I0868207

CCCN®

Exam

Practice Questions

Mometrix

TEST PREPARATION

DEAR FUTURE EXAM SUCCESS STORY

First of all, **THANK YOU** for purchasing Mometrix study materials!

Second, congratulations! You are one of the few determined test-takers who are committed to doing whatever it takes to excel on your exam. **You have come to the right place.** We developed these practice tests with one goal in mind: to deliver you the best possible approximation of the questions you will see on test day.

Standardized testing is one of the biggest obstacles on your road to success, which only increases the importance of doing well in the high-pressure, high-stakes environment of test day. Your results on this test could have a significant impact on your future, and these practice tests will give you the repetitions you need to build your familiarity and confidence with the test content and format to help you achieve your full potential on test day.

Your success is our success

We would love to hear from you! If you would like to share the story of your exam success or if you have any questions or comments in regard to our products, please contact us at **800-673-8175** or **support@mometrix.com**.

Thanks again for your business and we wish you continued success!

Sincerely,
The Mometrix Test Preparation Team

Written and edited by the Mometrix Exam Secrets Test Prep Team
Printed in the United States of America

TABLE OF CONTENTS

Practice Test #1

1. Considering the urgency wave perceived when a patient feels the need to urinate, which of the following is the best initial response to urgency?

a. sit down and stay still
b. do 5 quick flicks of the pelvic floor muscles
c. use distraction
d. walk slowly

2. Which of the following drugs is probably the best next choice for a patient who wants to discontinue oxybutynin ER because of severe dry mouth?

a. Trospium IR (20 mg BID)
b. Oxybutynin TDS (3.9 mg)
c. Darifenacin (15 mg)
d. Tolterodine ER (4 mg QID)

3. Constipation is usually defined as fewer than how many stools per week?

a. 7
b. 5
c. 3
d. 2

4. Slow-transit constipation is characterized by

a. difficulty defecating with straining but normal frequency.
b. reduced frequency of stools, reduced peristalsis, and abdominal distention.
c. normal frequency and difficulty defecating with some loose stools.
d. prolonged defecation (greater than 10 minutes) and need for rectal splinting.

5. What is the most common type of urinary incontinence?

a. urge
b. stress
c. mixed
d. functional

6. What are the 3 major physical consequences of incontinence?

a. skin breakdown, urinary tract infections, and depression
b. skin breakdown, confusion, and depression
c. skin breakdown, falls, and depression
d. skin breakdown, falls, and urinary tract infections

7. Chronic urinary retention is characterized by

a. painful bladder.
b. non-palpable distention.
c. non-painful bladder.
d. impaired fecal evaluation.

8. How much urine can usually be stored in the renal pelvis?

a. 10 to 15 mL
b. 15 to 30 mL
c. 30 to 45 mL
d. 45 to 60 mL

9. Which part of the female urethra serves as a sphincter mechanism?

a. proximal one-third
b. distal middle third
c. distal end third
d. entire urethra

10. When catheterizing a patient, what is the primary factor that allows drainage through the catheter while preventing leakage around the catheter?

a. size of catheter
b. size of urethra
c. urethral softness
d. urethral sphincter contraction

11. A patient with congestive heart failure and peripheral edema usually experiences

a. stress incontinence.
b. nocturia.
c. nocturnal enuresis.
d. functional incontinence.

12. In older adults, what is the primary difference between males and females with overactive bladder?

a. males have more bladder outlet obstruction
b. females have more bladder outlet obstruction
c. males experience more nocturia
d. females experience more nocturia

13. What is the pelvic organ prolapse that involves the anterior vaginal wall?

a. cystocele
b. uterine prolapse
c. vaginal vault prolapse
d. rectocele

14. What is the primary treatment for pelvic organ prolapse?

a. surgical repair
b. medication
c. manual reduction
d. pessary

15. What is the most common cause of encopresis?

a. behavioral problem
b. psychological disorder
c. chronic constipation
d. anatomic abnormalities

16. Which of the following is most indicated for an inactive patient who has been taking laxatives long-term to treat chronic bouts of constipation and fecal impaction?

a. stool softeners
b. high-fiber diet
c. exercise program
d. bowel retraining

17. Which of the following tests used to assess cognitive abilities for a patient with dementia includes remembering and later repeating the names of 3 common objects and drawing the face of a clock with all 12 number and the hands indicating a specified time?

a. Mini-cog
b. Mini-mental state exam (MMSE)
c. Instrumental Activities of Daily Living (IADL)
d. Confusion Assessment Method

18. What is the primary purpose of conducting a bedside ultrasound bladder scan?

a. to diagnose structural abnormalities of the urinary system
b. to diagnose bladder tumors
c. to guide catheter placement
d. to assess urinary volume/retention

19. When evaluating a patient's home environment for safety issues, which of the following is of most concern for a patient who has an unstable gait and uses a gliding walker to navigate to the bathroom?

a. there are 4 cats and 2 dogs in the home
b. the kitchen is poorly lit
c. there are numerous loose rugs and piles of papers strewn about on the floors
d. the bathroom lacks grab bars

20. Which of the following is the best solution for a patient with moderately severe dementia of the Alzheimer type who is incontinent of urine during the daytime and at night?

a. scheduled toileting every 2 hours during the daytime
b. indwelling catheter (Foley)
c. clean intermittent catheterization
d. absorbent undergarments

21. If, during the abdominal exam, percussion of a protuberant abdomen exhibits a tympanitic percussion note, this probably indicates

a. gaseous distention.
b. fat deposits.
c. solid tumor.
d. ascitic fluid.

22. Small, round, firm, yellow nodules with black centers noted on the labia are probably

a. epidermoid cysts.
b. venereal warts.
c. genital herpes.
d. carcinoma.

23. On pelvic exam, the nurse notes an irregular cauliflower-appearing lesion on the cervix, which is most likely

a. cervical polyp.
b. cervical carcinoma.
c. retention cyst.
d. mucopurulent cervicitis.

24. On rectal exam of a female patient, a firm rectal shelf felt behind the cervix and uterus in the rectouterine pouch usually indicates

a. internal hemorrhoids.
b. external hemorrhoids.
c. peritoneal metastasis.
d. polyps.

25. If an 80-year-old woman has no response to the anal wink test or bulbocavernosus reflex, this probably indicates

a. impaired sacral nerve reflexes.
b. normal variation.
c. neurological disease.
d. neurogenic bladder.

26. For the most effective prevention of childbirth-related urinary incontinence, the woman should practice pelvic floor exercises throughout

a. pregnancy and the post-partum period.
b. the second trimester and the post-partum period.
c. the third trimester and the post-partum period.
d. the postpartum period only.

27. Which of the following is a normal age-related change to the urinary system?

a. faster awareness of the urge to urinate
b. fewer uninhibited contractions of the detrusor muscle
c. decreased contractility of the detrusor muscle
d. urethra lengthens

28. Postvoid/terminal voiding occurs most often in women when they

a. exit the bathroom.
b. rise from the toilet.
c. bend over shortly after urination.
d. sit down shortly after urination.

29. The primary reason that people fail to seek medical help for urinary incontinence is the erroneous belief that

a. no treatment is available.
b. urinary incontinence is shameful.
c. individuals can manage urinary incontinence without medical assistance.
d. incontinence is part of normal aging.

30. When reviewing a patient's bladder diary, the most important element of assessment is determining

a. frequency.
b. intake.
c. patterns.
d. amount of incontinence.

31. Which of the following should a patient with an overactive bladder avoid?

a. coffee
b. milk
c. bananas
d. carrots

32. Dependent continence means that the patient

a. is sometimes continent, depending on the circumstances.
b. depends on absorbent products to contain incontinence.
c. is kept free of incontinence through effort of caregivers.
d. must restrict fluid to remain continent.

33. A patient with advanced Parkinson's disease is most likely to experience

a. stress incontinence.
b. urge incontinence.
c. urinary retention.
d. decreased bladder capacity.

34. When removing a silicone Gellhorn pessary, if the pessary will not rotate or move with the tenaculum forceps and the nurse cannot digitally break the seal, what is the next step?

a. do a vaginal irrigation
b. change patient's position
c. apply external traction to the knob
d. inject normal saline through the opening in the pessary

35. The most common indication of prostatic cancer is

a. pain.
b. increasing signs of urinary obstruction.
c. increasing urinary incontinence.
d. onset of fecal incontinence.

36. When conducting medication reconciliation, the nurse finds the patient's list of current medications includes furosemide, metolazone, dioctyl calcium sulfosuccinate and docusate calcium, with prescriptions from two physicians. What does this probably indicate?

a. polypharmacy
b. inaccurate reporting
c. good medical management
d. negligent medical management

37. Which of the following is a best practice for bladder retraining with catheter removal?

a. administer antibiotic prophylaxis
b. schedule routine clamping of the catheter prior to removal
c. schedule timed voiding
d. palpate bladder after urination to evaluate urinary retention

38. Which of the following interventions is most appropriate for a 35-year-old woman with multiple sclerosis having recurrent episodes of constipation but only rare fecal incontinence?

a. laxatives PRN for constipation
b. nutritional assessment
c. daily glycerine suppository
d. bowel training

39. Which vaginal pH is consistent with adequate estrogen?

a. 4.8
b. 5.6
c. 6
d. 7

40. When adjusting the duty cycle for pelvic floor electrical stimulation, which ratio of stimulation to non-stimulation is usually most appropriate for an initial setting?

a. 2:1
b. 1:1
c. 3:1
d. 1:2

41. When a patient is practicing pelvic floor muscle (Kegel) exercises in the reclining position, the knees should be bent and supported in order to

a. increase pressure on the pelvic floor muscles.
b. prevent backache.
c. prevent tightening of thigh muscles.
d. reduce the urge to urinate.

42. If a patient's bladder capacity is about 300 mL and the patient's output is approximately 1300 to 1500 mL daily, how many times should the patient schedule clean intermittent catheterization each day?

a. 2 to 3 times
b. 5 to 6 times
c. 8 to 10 times
d. 12 times

43. What is the most likely initial treatment for a patient with post-prostatectomy incontinence characterized by frequency, enuresis, and urge incontinence?

a. anticholinergics
b. bladder pacemaker
c. artificial urinary sphincter
d. male urethral sling procedure

44. When assessing bladder capacity, functional capacity refers to the volume of urine the bladder

a. is able to hold during urodynamic studies.
b. is able to hold when the patient is anesthetized or sedated.
c. expels during urination.
d. can hold before sensations of urgency occur.

45. Which type of urinary incontinence is most likely to occur at night when the patient is lying in supine position?

a. overflow incontinence
b. urge incontinence
c. stress incontinence
d. mixed incontinence

46. With uroflowmetry, when evaluating the normal flow pattern, the maximum or peak flow per second is generally defined as

a. greater than 15 mL.
b. 10-15 mL.
c. less than 10 mL.
d. 5 mL.

47. Urethral pressure profile and the maximum urethral closure pressure (MUCP) are usually measured with what?

a. standard straight catheter
b. transducer
c. ultrasound
d. electromyogram

48. When conducting electromyogram using skin surface sensors about the anus, at what clock position are the electrodes usually placed?

a. 12 and 6 o'clock
b. 12, 4, and 8 o'clock
c. 10 and 4 o'clock
d. 3 and 9 o'clock

49. Following a cystoscopy, what is the most common adverse effect?

a. hypotension
b. bleeding
c. dysuria
d. infection

50. When conducting the Q-tip test, which change in angle indicates urethral hypermobility?

a. 10 degrees
b. greater than 20 degrees
c. greater than 30 degrees
d. greater than 45 degrees

51. When undergoing a bowel transit time test, how soon after ingesting markers should the patient return for radiographs?

a. 24 hours
b. 2 days
c. 4 days
d. 5 days

52. What is the function of the rectoanal inhibitory reflex?

a. relax the internal anal sphincter
b. relax the external anal sphincter
c. contract the internal anal sphincter
d. contract the external anal sphincter

53. What is the most common cause of fecal incontinence?

a. chronic diarrhea
b. fecal impaction
c. neurological impairment
d. laxative abuse

54. The purpose of the balloon expulsion test is to evaluate

a. general ability to defecate.
b. internal and external sphincters.
c. rectal sensation.
d. nerve damage.

55. Which of the following is a bowel irritant that may cause or increase diarrhea?

a. cheese
b. applesauce
c. caffeine
d. carbonated beverage

56. When considering the waist-to-hip ratio (waist measurement divided by hip measurement), which of the following indicates high risk of obesity-related health problems for a female?

a. 0.81 to 0.85
b. greater than 0.85
c. 0.9 to 0.95
d. greater than 1.0

57. During the provocative stress (cough) test, what is the minimum volume of urine that the bladder should contain?

a. 50 mL
b. 100 mL
c. 150 mL
d. 200 mL

58. Which is usually the preferred method of fluid modification for an older adult with nocturia?

a. restrict overall fluid intake
b. continue normal fluid intake in the morning and afternoon and restrict fluids after 6 PM
c. continue normal fluid intake in the morning and restrict fluids after 2 PM
d. increase fluid intake in the morning and afternoon and restrict fluids after 6 PM

59. During bladder training, a crucial component is teaching the patient about

a. mechanics of urination.
b. distraction and relaxation techniques.
c. fluid modification.
d. diet modifications.

60. Obsessive toileting is usually caused by

a. urinary infection.
b. cognitive impairment.
c. fear of incontinence.
d. psychiatric disorder.

61. When using posterior tibial nerve stimulation (PTNS) for treatment of urge incontinence, correct needle placement is verified by

a. the great toe bending downward.
b. the great toe bending upward.
c. the second toe bending upward.
d. the toes feeling numb.

62. Which of the following patients most at risk for functional incontinence?

a. patients with severe depression
b. patients who are frail and elderly
c. patients with cognitive impairment
d. patients with impaired mobility

63. Patients with spinal shock after a spinal cord injury are most at risk for

a. detrusor overactivity.
b. bladder outlet obstruction.
c. detrusor-sphincter dyssynergia.
d. atonic bladder.

64. Which of the following is the greatest risk factor for the development of bladder cancer?

a. African American race
b. smoking
c. female gender
d. chronic cystitis

65. When evaluating renal function in an older adult to determine how well a drug will be metabolized, the best laboratory assessment is the

a. blood, urea, nitrogen (BUN).
b. creatinine clearance.
c. serum creatinine.
d. urinalysis.

66. When evaluating an older adult's functional mobility, which of the following is a safe maneuver?

a. supporting the leg and pushing the knee into flexion
b. asking the patient to hop on one foot
c. asking the patient to do deep knee bends
d. supporting the arm and asking the patient to flex the elbow

67. Which of the following sports activities may increase risk of stress urinary incontinence?

a. volleyball
b. swimming
c. walking
d. bicycling

68. When a male patient is considering use of a penile clamp to control urinary incontinence, the most important factor to assess is

a. the degree of urinary leakage.
b. penile sensation.
c. penile length.
d. penile circumference.

69. What is the normal transit time of stool through the colon?

a. 12 to 24 hours
b. 24 to 48 hours
c. 36 to 72 hours
d. 72 to 96 hours

70. An enterocele involves herniation of the

a. vagina.
b. bladder.
c. urethra.
d. uterus.

71. What is the most common physiological result of menopause?

a. thickening of the skin
b. atrophic vaginitis
c. bacterial vaginitis
d. recurrent urine infection

72. What is the most common organism cultured from patients with a first incidence of urinary infection?

a. *Staphylococcus aureus*
b. *Pseudomonas aeruginosa*
c. β-Streptococcus
d. *Escherichia coli*

73. Which of the following drugs is usually recommended for urogenital atrophy in females?

a. transvaginal estrogen
b. oral estrogen
c. duloxetine
d. bethanechol

74. Which of the following urinary incontinence devices is probably the best choice for an elderly male who occasionally dribbles small amounts of urine and who favors loose boxer shorts?

a. guard leaf-shaped pad
b. perineal pad
c. protective underwear
d. drip collector sock

75. When choosing an absorbent incontinent product, what is the best absorbent padding?

a. cotton
b. paper
c. superabsorbent polymer
d. polyester

76. Which of the following catheter types is the best choice for long-term indwelling catheterization for urinary retention?

a. latex
b. Teflon-coated latex
c. silicone-coated latex
d. silicone (100%)

77. Daily meatal or catheter insertion site care for a patient with an indwelling catheter should include use of

a. povidone-iodine.
b. soap and water.
c. antibacterial cream/ointment.
d. hydrogen peroxide.

78. With the five-point (0 to 5) Baden-Walker grading scale for pelvic organ prolapse, a uterine prolapse that extends halfway down the vagina toward the hymen (opening) would be classified as what grade?

a. grade 1
b. grade 2
c. grade 3
d. grade 4

79. What is the most common surgical procedure to treat stress urinary incontinence?

a. Burch colposuspension
b. Marshall-Marchetti-Krantz bladder neck suspension
c. bladder augmentation
d. midurethral sling

80. What is the most common method that women with moderate to severe urinary incontinence use to avoid incontinence during sexual activity?

a. female condom
b. pre-coital urination
c. abstinence
d. diaphragm

81. If teaching a patient with spinal cord injury to do digital stimulation, the patient should be advised that once the rectum starts to empty, the patient should continue the stimulation

a. for five minutes.
b. for 1 minute.
c. during the entire defecation.
d. during the entire defecation and for 5 additional minutes.

82. If a patient has recently developed intermittent fecal incontinence, the first step in developing patient-centered goals for continence is to

a. assess the patient's for normal defecation pattern.
b. review the patient's lists of medications.
c. assess the condition of the patient's perineal skin.
d. review fluid and food intake.

83. If a patient is undergoing bowel training in the morning after breakfast with a bisacodyl suppository, how frequently should digital stimulation be carried out after the suppository is inserted?

a. once in 5 minutes if no evacuation.
b. every 2 to 3 minutes until evacuation.
c. every 10 to 15 minutes until evacuation.
d. after initial evacuation to ensure rectum has emptied.

84. If a patient has a urethral insert (FemSoft®) and has inserted it with a stylus in place, how should the patient remove the insert?

a. reinsert the stylus and press inward to flatten the balloon and then pull out
b. gently pull straight outward on the insert
c. reinsert the stylus and push forward until no resistance is felt and balloon is punctured
d. pull downward on the insert

85. For a male patient to safely use a penile compression device, such as a penile clamp, the patient must

a. have normal vision.
b. have normal sensation.
c. limit use to one hour daily.
d. have assistance in use.

86. If a patient has developed urinary incontinence but it's unclear if it is a transient problem, the first step should be to

a. keep a 3-day bladder/bowel record.
b. begin a trial of bladder training.
c. begin a trial of prompted voiding.
d. begin a trial of scheduled toileting.

87. Biofeedback with a pressure-sensitive probe inserted into the rectum is likely to be most effective for fecal incontinence associated with

a. absence of rectal sensation.
b. underlying neurological disease.
c. psychological-associated incontinence.
d. weak sphincter muscles.

88. Which of the following may indicate recruitment of additional muscle groups when assessing a patient trying to contract pelvic floor muscles during pelvic floor muscle training?

a. pressing heels to the floor
b. expiring heavily
c. holding breath
d. relaxing arm muscles

89. A poorly-controlled diabetic patient has had frequent fecal impaction with overflow fecal incontinence because of chronic constipation that results from

a. the kidneys drawing water as a solvent for unmetabolized sugar.
b. impaired ability of the bowels to reabsorb liquids.
c. lack of sensation of thirst with resultant dehydration.
d. inadequate fiber in a diabetic diet.

90. When teaching a male patient to use a reusable external condom catheter, how often should the nurse advise the patient to remove the external catheter for cleaning?

a. every 8 hours
b. every 12 hours
c. every 24 hours
d. every 48 hours

91. If an indwelling urinary catheter has been in place for 2 weeks and the patient's urine is cloudy, in order to obtain a urine specimen for culture and sensitivities, the nurse should

a. disconnect the catheter from tubing and collect specimen directly from the catheter.
b. flush the catheter with NS and wait 20 minutes to collect the specimen directly from the catheter.
c. collect the specimen directly from the drainage bag.
d. change the catheter and collect specimen directly from the new catheter.

92. Which of the following is the most appropriate management product for a nonambulatory patient with dementia with moderate to heavy urinary incontinence?

a. X-large underpads
b. indwelling catheter
c. pull-on disposable incontinence briefs
d. adjustable disposable incontinence briefs with Velcro closings

93. Which diagnostic study is most effective in diagnosing the type of urinary incontinence a patient is experiencing?

a. videourodynamic studies
b. cystoscopy
c. ultrasound
d. CT scan

94. Pessaries are most likely to become dislodged during

a. walking and bending.
b. urination and defecation.
c. sexual intercourse.
d. sleeping.

95. Which of the following may increase the adverse effects of oxybutynin?

a. antacids
b. dairy products
c. tomatoes
d. grapefruit

96. If a 64-year-old female patient has persistent overflow incontinence because of an areflexic detrusor muscle, the recommended treatment is

a. urinary diversion.
b. Foley catheter.
c. clean intermittent catheterization.
d. protective pads.

97. Which of the following is the most important factor in determining whether an event is a stressor to a patient?

a. patient's education
b. patient age
c. patient's perception
d. patient's support system

98. If a woman with an overactive bladder is concerned about leaking urine during sexual intercourse and has avoided sexual intimacy, the best advice is to

a. take steps to minimize leakage.
b. stop worrying about it.
c. continue to avoid sexual intimacy.
d. avoid all liquids for 6 to 8 hours before intimacy.

99. If a patient is undergoing the stage one trial period with the InterStim® sacral nerve stimulator, which of the following is considered a successful response?

a. >30% decrease in number of voids per day
b. >40% increase in volume of voids
c. >40% decrease in number of catheterizations per day
d. >50% decrease in number of leaking episodes per day

100. The most effective position for active listening is

a. sitting beside the patient, touching the patient's arm.
b. standing near the patient with arms uncrossed.
c. sitting directly in front of patient with arms uncrossed.
d. any position because position is irrelevant.

101. Which of the following is a nonverbal clue that a patient may be anxious?

a. patient rubs eyes and yawns
b. patient has flat aspect and responds in monosyllables
c. patient pupils are constricted and patient sniffs repeatedly
d. patient rubs hands together constantly

102. Which of the following is most likely to cover the costs of incontinent supplies (such as absorbant pads and adult diapers) at no cost to patients?

a. Medicare
b. Medicaid
c. private insurance
d. manufacturers

103. A female patient with urinary incontinence reports that she feels less physically attractive and more dissatisfied with her body and finds it difficult to look at herself naked although other aspects of her life are good, this suggests

a. depression.
b. impaired body image.
c. ambivalence.
d. confusion.

104. If the nurse hears a patient's physician complaining that a patient is "difficult and impatient," and the nurse tells the physician that the patient is very frightened and acting defensively, the aspect of care that the nurse is exhibiting is

a. advocacy.
b. patient equality.
c. human dignity preservation.
d. caring practice.

105. If a female patient is scheduled for a sling procedure to correct stress incontinence, the patient should be advised to avoid sexual intercourse postoperatively for at least

a. 2 weeks.
b. 4 weeks.
c. 6 weeks.
d. 8 weeks.

106. When applying no-sting barrier film (such as Cavilon™ spray) to protect the skin from urinary or fecal incontinence, the spay container should be held

a. 2 to 3 inches above the skin.
b. 4 to 6 inches above the skin.
c. 7 to 9 inches above the skin.
d. 10 to 12 inches above the skin.

107. Which of the following is the least effective in protecting the skin from incontinence-associated dermatitis?

a. zinc oxide
b. petrolatum
c. soap and water
d. lanolin

108. If a patient has developed low anterior resection syndrome with persistent fecal incontinence of semi-solid stool, which of the following may help to reduce the incontinence?

a. Imodium AD
b. increased intake of dairy products
c. limit fluid intake
d. Kegel exercises and dietary modifications

109. If an older adult has sudden onset of confusion and urinary incontinence, and slight unsteadiness but has no complaints of dysuria, the nurse should suspect

a. stroke.
b. urinary tract infection.
c. dementia.
d. diabetes.

110. Which of the following is a risk factor for development of a cystocele?

a. obesity
b. multiple sex partners
c. history of STDs
d. history of Cesarean

111. Which of the following foods should be avoided for those with overactive bladder?

a. dairy products
b. starchy foods
c. spicy foods
d. cruciferous vegetables

112. OnabotulinumtoxinA (Botox®) has been approved by the FDA for treatment of

a. stress incontinence.
b. fecal incontinence.
c. overflow incontinence.
d. overactive bladder.

113. Which type of pessary may be utilized for treatment of a mild rectocele?

a. Gelhorn
b. Gehrung
c. donut
d. hodge

114. If a patient with overactive bladder reports that she has severely limited fluids in order to decrease incontinence, the nurse should advise the patient that

a. this may increase bladder irritation.
b. this is an effective method.
c. this will likely have no effect.
d. this may cause serious adverse effects.

115. When assessing vaginal pH during a pelvic exam, what vaginal pH is consistent with atrophic vaginitis?

a. 4 to 4.8
b. 4.8 to 5
c. 5 to 5.4
d. 5.5 to 7

116. The first step in prompted voiding is

a. prompting.
b. talking.
c. checking.
d. praising.

117. If a patient with venous insufficiency tends to develop peripheral edema by evening and this corresponds with nocturia, the patient should be advised to

a. take diuretics in the morning rather than at night.
b. decrease fluid intake throughout the day.
c. avoid all sodium-containing foods.
d. wear compression stockings and elevate feet/legs in the afternoon/evening.

118. Which of the following conditions is commonly associated with tenesmus and fecal urgency?

a. ulcerative proctitis
b. internal hemorrhoids
c. anal fissure
d. Crohn's disease

119. With the Q-tip urethral test, the angle of the Q-tip with straining or coughing that corresponds to urethral hypermobility is

a. ≥45 degrees.
b. ≤45 degrees.
c. ≥30 degrees.
d. ≤30 degrees.

120. If utilizing double voiding for urinary retention, the patient should urinate and then

a. remain seated and urinate again in 2 to 10 minutes.
b. remain seated and urinate again in one minute.
c. get up and move about for 5 minutes and then urinate again.
d. get up and move about for 15 minutes and then urinate again.

Answers and Explanations

1. A: The urgency wave is like a Bell curve. First the person feels an urge, which then grows and peaks before subsiding and stopping. The best initial response to the feeling of urgency is to sit down and stay still, breathing slowly and deeply. The next step is to do 5 quick flicks (2-3 seconds duration each) of the pelvic floor muscles, and then use distraction, which can include relaxation exercises and self-affirming statements. The patient should try to wait a few minutes to see if the urge subsides and then, if necessary, walk slowly to the toilet.

2. B: Dry mouth and constipation are the two most common adverse effects of anti-muscarinic drugs used to treat overactive bladder. Dry mouth occurs in up to 61% of those taking oxybutynin ER, but oxybutynin TDS, the transdermal patch, has a much lower incidence, ranging from about 4% to 10%. Darifenacin has incidence of about 35% and tolterodine ER of about 23%. Thus, oxybutynin TDS is probably the best choice. Additionally, compliance with transdermal patches is usually better than with oral medications. Oxybutynin TDS is applied twice weekly.

3. C: Constipation is usually defined as fewer than 3 stools per week although there is considerable individual variation. Some people have 2 to 3 stools daily while others only defecate every 2 or 3 days, so it's necessary to determine the normal pattern for a patient when assessing constipation. Constipation is also sometimes described in terms of stool consistency (hard, small) and difficulty defecating (need to strain, splinting). Constipation is most common in patients in their 60s, with rates about 5 times those of younger adults.

4. B: Slow-transit constipation: Reduced frequency of stools to less than or equal to 1 time weekly because of decreased peristalsis. Patients may experience abdominal distention and discomfort. Normal transit constipation: Normal frequency but difficulty defecating, requiring straining, but no loose stools. Rectosigmoidal constipation: Involves outlet obstruction and inability to relax muscles involved in defecation, so defecation is often prolonged greater than 10 minutes and frequency is reduced. The patient often must use anal stimulation or splinting to aid evacuation. Stool may become very hard.

5. B: Stress incontinence is the most common type of incontinence. While statistics have varied, most studies indicate that at least 50% of incontinence is stress incontinence; however, there are some variations according to age and condition. Younger adults (primarily women) tend to have more stress incontinence, but older adults tend to have more urge incontinence and mixed incontinence. Functional incontinence is a factor in those with chronic health conditions, such as arthritis and Parkinson disease, and may combine with other types of incontinence.

6. D: The 3 major physical consequences of incontinence are skin breakdown, falls, and urinary tract infections. Incontinence can lead to maceration of the skin and, combined with immobility, increases the risk of developing pressure injuries. Up to 8 in 10 elderly adults experience nocturia, and many leak urine on the way to the toilet, increasing the risk of falls. Urinary tract infections are common in those with incontinence, with both absorptive products and catheterization increasing risk.

7. C: Both acute and chronic urinary retention are characterized by distended bladder that is palpable and percussible, but acute retention is associated with pain and the inability to urinate. Those with chronic urinary retention become desensitized and no longer experience pain. Thus, chronic urinary retention tends to correspond with overflow incontinence, as patients may be less aware of the need to urinate. With chronic urinary retention, the patient is able to urinate, but urination is inadequate, and the bladder remains distended after urination.

8. B: The renal pelvis, where transportation of the urine occurs, can store 15 to 30 mL of urine. The renal pelvis connects with the ureters at the ureteropelvic junction. Urine flows from the renal pelvis to the ureters and bladder by peristaltic action as the pelvis fills, propelling between 5 and 15 mL of urine at low pressure down the ureters and into the bladder. Any condition that increases pressure, such as outlet obstruction, may interfere with this transportation system and result in renal damage.

9. D: The female urethra is usually about 3.5 to 5.5 cm long, and almost the entire length of the urethra acts as a sphincter mechanism. The male urethra is about 23 cm long and has two distinct functional sections, the proximal and the distal. The proximal portion, which extends through the prostate and has 3 parts (proximal, prostatic, and membranous urethra), forms the sphincter mechanism while the distal portion serves only as an outlet for urine.

10. C: Urethral softness is the ability of the urethra to change shape in order to create a seal to prevent leakage and then to relax and allow urination. When a catheter is passed through the urethra, this factor allows the urethra to conform to the shape of the catheter, allowing drainage while sealing around the catheter to prevent leakage. However, trauma from long-term catheterization or repeat catheterizations can impair the ability of the urethra to form a tight seal, resulting in persistent leakage even with a large-sized catheter.

11. B: Nocturia (typically two to three times nightly) occurs with CHF and peripheral edema. This is because dependency during daytime hours increases edema, which decreases when the legs are elevated during sleep, and the extra fluid is filtered through the kidneys at night. Most CHF patients take diuretics, which also increase nocturia. Additionally, older adults, on average, produce about 50% of their urinary output during the night, whereas younger adults produce most of their urine output during the daytime.

12. A: The primary difference between older males and females with overactive bladder is that males tend to have more bladder outlet obstruction than females. Overactive bladder in males is commonly associated with benign prostatic hypertrophy, occurring in about 50% of those with BPH. BPH typically results in bladder outlet obstruction, although whether the overactive bladder is a direct result of BPH is not clear. Overactive bladder with incontinence increases markedly in males after age 40 and continues to increase with age with prevalence of overactive bladder and urge incontinence much higher in males than females.

13. A: Cystocele: This prolapse is of the anterior vaginal wall and bladder into the vagina. This is the most common type of prolapse.

Uterine prolapse: This prolapse is of the cervix and neck of the uterus into the vagina.

Vaginal vault prolapse: Weakness of the apex of the vagina causes it to evert and prolapse distally through the vagina.

Rectocele: This prolapse is of the posterior vaginal wall and rectum into the vagina.

14. D: The pessary is the primary treatment for pelvic organ prolapse. Pessaries are plastic or silicone removable prosthetic devices that are placed in the vagina for treatment of pelvic organ prolapse as well as stress incontinence. There are a wide variety of pessaries, and they are fitted to the individual. A pelvic exam is done prior to fitting a person for a pessary. Fitting sets are available to help the healthcare provider pick the right size, as the correct fit is crucial if the pessary is to be comfortable and provide needed support.

15. C: Retentive encopresis (80%) is characterized by a history of long-term, painful constipation and the development of overflow diarrhea. The chronic constipation causes distention of the rectum and stretching of both the internal and external anal sphincters, so the child may no longer feel the urge to defecate, and stool eventually leaks from the rectum. Non-retentive encopresis (20%), usually involving passage of normally formed stools on a daily basis, does not involve constipation or bowel abnormalities, except in a small subset that may have irritable bowel syndrome, but is generally a behavioral/psychological problem.

16. D: Bowel retraining strategies include:

- Keeping a bowel diary for a week.
- Modifying diet and fluid intake to assure normal stool consistency, including increased fiber and fluids, eating meals at scheduled times, and avoiding foods that increase bowel dysfunction.
- Establishing a schedule for defecation, preferably at the same time each day and about 20-30 minutes after a meal.
- Practicing Kegel exercises.
- Using a stimulus to promote defecation, such as enemas, suppositories, or laxatives in the beginning, with a goal to decrease such use. Digital stimulation or hot drinks may be used.
- Keeping a record of stool consistency and evacuation.

17. A: The Mini-cog test requires the person to remember and later repeat the names of 3 common objects and to draw the face of a clock with all 12 numbers and 2 hands indicated a specified time. The MMSE requires a number of tasks, including counting backward from 100 by 7s, providing current location, repeating phrases, following directions, and copying a picture of interlocking shapes. IADL measure 8 activities necessary for adults to function independently (including shopping, food preparation, telephone use, and managing finances). The Confusion Assessment Method is used to assess development of delirium, not dementia.

18. D: The ultrasound bladder scan is most often used to assess urinary volume and urinary retention. For example, it may be used after urination to evaluate residual urine rather than using catheterization. The scan may also be used to verify the need for catheterization by assessing urine volume or bladder distension. The goals associated with using the bladder scan include decreasing the need for catheterization and thereby decreasing incidence of urinary infections, decreasing costs, and increasing patient comfort.

19. C: Environmental hazards such as piles of papers or junk on the floors, loose carpet or rugs, and cluttered pathways can cause falls and must be cleared, organized, or repaired because they pose an immediate risk to a person with an unstable gait who must use a walker. Animals may pose a danger, depending on how well trained or cared for they are. They should have access to food, water, toileting, and routine veterinary care. Lighting should be adequate enough for reading in all rooms and stairways. Bathrooms may require grab bars, hand-held shower, and elevated toilet or tub seats.

20. D: The best solution for patients with moderate to severe dementia of the Alzheimer type and urinary incontinence is absorbent undergarments, although keeping them on patients can prove challenging. They do increase the risk of urinary tract infection, so they must be changed frequently and the patient's skin cleansed thoroughly. If irritation occurs, a skin barrier should be applied.

Scheduled toileting may reduce incontinence, but some patients lose awareness of urination or are confused about the function of a toilet. Patients often pull out Foley catheters and resist catheterization.

21. A: Gaseous distention: Results in a tympanitic percussion note. The gaseous distention may be localized to one area of the bowel or generalized. Distention may result from eating some foods or may indicate blockage. Gaseous distention is greater with colonic obstruction than with small bowel obstruction. Fat deposits: Results in normal percussive note. Solid tumor: Results in dull percussive note, similar to a severely distended bladder. Ascitic fluid: Results in dull percussive note with shift in location if patient's position changed.

22. A: Small (2 to 5 mm), round, firm, cystic yellow or white nodules, sometimes with black centers (from blocked duct), located on the labia majora or minora are probably epidermoid cysts. Epidermoid cysts may become infected and painful with erythema, edema, and purulent discharge, but they are usually benign and quite common in older females. Epidermoid cysts usually require no treatment although they can be surgically removed if necessary. Good hygiene is essential to preventing infection.

23. B: Early stages of cervical carcinoma may be difficult to detect visually, but in the advanced stages, cervical carcinoma may appear as an irregular, fungating, cauliflower-appearing mass. Most cases of cervical carcinoma are associated with human papillomavirus infection. Most of those with cervical carcinoma are younger than 55 years of age. Treatment depends on staging and the age of the patient but can include surgery (especially for stages 1 and 2), radiation, and/or chemotherapy. Radiation and chemotherapy are often indicated if the cancer has spread beyond the cervix.

24. C: Palpating a firm rectal shelf behind the cervix and uterus in the rectouterine pouch usually indicates peritoneal metastasis, which may originate from various sources. Internal hemorrhoids are usually not palpable until they prolapse, at which point they appear red and moist and may be accompanied by bleeding. External hemorrhoids are visible swollen, blue-tinged masses covered with skin. Polyps are quite soft and often difficult to reach or palpate, so proctoscopy or colonoscopy is usually required to identify.

25. B: Older females often have no response to the anal wink test, and up to 20% of women also do not exhibit the bulbocavernosus reflex. So, these tests are inconclusive, and the results are a normal variation for women. The anal wink test, elicited by stroking the tissue about the anus, evaluates the S2 to S4 sacral reflexes. The bulbocavernosus reflex test, elicited by gently squeezing the clitoris in females and the glans penis in males, also tests the S2 to S4 sacral reflexes and is often used to evaluate innervation of the perineal striated muscles.

26. A: While practicing pelvic floor exercises is beneficial at any stage of pregnancy, even if started postpartum, ideally instructions regarding exercises should be given prepartum and the woman should continue with the exercises throughout pregnancy and during the postpartum period. This decreases incontinence during the last trimester and after delivery. Studies have shown that the woman needs to do at least 28 contractions daily to receive benefit. Vaginal delivery is one of the leading causes of urinary incontinence in females although increased risk also occurs with Cesarean.

27. C: A number of normal changes in the urinary system occur with age, including decreased contractility of the detrusor muscle because of muscular atrophy, which prevents the bladder from completely emptying and increasing the need to urinate more frequently. Other changes include slowing of sensory awareness of the urge to urinate, so people are less able to delay urination.

Detrusor hyperactivity increases the frequency of the urge to urinate, and the urethra tends to shorten. Bladder capacity itself normally remains the same unless there is an abnormality.

28. B: Postvoid or terminal voiding, intermittent dribbling or loss of urine shortly after urination, occurs most often in women when they rise from the toilet and often results in soiling of undergarments and clothes. Because men usually urinate standing, they tend to experience the dribbling of urine as they exit the bathroom. The most common cause is urinary retention that results in the bladder staying partially full. In females, urethral diverticulum may also be a cause.

29. D: Since urinary incontinence is so common, especially in women who have experienced childbirth, many patients believe that incontinence is part of normal aging and something that they simply have to live with. Aside from feelings of shame, many patients also are unaware that effective treatments are available, so they alter their lifestyles to accommodate their incontinence instead of seeking medical help. Some people become increasingly withdrawn and avoid social situations because of the fear of odor or incontinence.

30. C: While all of these are important elements to consider, the most important element is determining patterns—when the patient tends to have incontinence (day and/or night), the relationship to fluid intake, frequency—because this can help to develop a plan to deal with the incontinence. The bladder diary should be kept for 3 to 5 days and should include time of incontinence and urination, amount of urination (small, medium, large), intake, estimated amount of incontinence, activity at time of incontinence, and sensation of urge.

31. A: A patient with an overactive bladder should avoid foods and beverages that are bladder irritants, such as all caffeinated products, including coffee, tea, chocolate, and some drugs (especially those containing caffeine, such as Anacin). Other foods to avoid include artificial sweeteners (such as aspartame and saccharine), highly acidic foods (such as citrus fruits) and highly spiced foods (especially those containing chili peppers, horseradish, spices, or hot sauces, such as Mexican, Indian, and Szechuan).

32. C: Dependent continence means that the patient has cognitive or physical impairment that prevents the person from controlling his/her own continence, but the patient is able to stay continent through the efforts of others. Without help, the patient would resume being incontinent or become incontinent. Care can include a caregiver who assists the patient to use the toilet or who maintains scheduled toileting. Dependent continence can also include those who are dependent on medications to prevent incontinence.

33. B: Parkinson's disease is a chronic progressive neurodegenerative disease that affects movement. Up to 70% of patients with advanced Parkinson's disease experience urinary dysfunction with detrusor overactivity, most often urgency, urge incontinence, frequency, and nocturia. Both voluntary and involuntary muscle control may be compromised, sometimes resulting in loss of sphincter control (especially of the rectal sphincter) and fecal incontinence. Additionally, muscle rigidity and impaired mobility may result in functional incontinence.

34. D: The soft silicone Gellhorn pessary is a concave disk with a stem with a knob. A small hole extends through the middle of the stem and the disk. Gellhorn is one of the most difficult pessaries to insert and remove as it is suctioned against the cervix or anterior vaginal wall (if cervix has been removed). The pessary is usually removed by grasping with forceps and rotating to break the seal. The seal may also be broken by inserting a finger behind the disk. If unsuccessful, normal saline can be injected through the center hole with a 50 mL syringe.

35. B: Indications of prostatic cancer are very nonspecific and similar to benign prostatic hypertrophy with increasing signs of urinary obstruction, including hesitancy, urgency, urinary retention, and nocturia. An elevated PSA test is one indication of prostatic cancer but is not conclusive, so transrectal biopsy is usually done to confirm the diagnosis with up to 10 biopsy samples taken from different areas of the prostate. In some cases, a diagnosis of prostatic cancer is made based on PSA and biopsy before the onset of symptoms.

36. A: Since furosemide and metolazone are both diuretics and dioctyl calcium sulfosuccinate and docusate calcium are both stool softeners, this list probably indicates polypharmacy. Older adults are especially at risk for polypharmacy, taking too many drugs, because of taking the same drug under generic and brand names, taking drugs for one condition that are contraindicated for another, and taking drugs that are not compatible. Reasons for polypharmacy include multiple prescriptions from different doctors; forgetfulness; confusion; failure to report current medications; the use of supplemental, over-the-counter, and herbal preparations in addition to prescribed medications; and failure of health care providers to adequately educate the patient.

37. C: Patients should have scheduled timed voiding after catheter removal, usually beginning with every 2 hours during the daytime. Best practices include avoiding the use of antibiotic prophylaxis unless evidence of bacteriuria persists at least 48 hours after a catheter is removed, and clamping is no longer advised before removing a catheter since it does not improve the ability to urinate and may result in reflux or bladder distention. Palpation of the bladder is not adequate to determine if urinary retention is present. For a few days after removal (and longer for some patients), residual urine should be checked with bladder ultrasound.

38. D: A comprehensive bowel-training program is often necessary for those with MS because about 70 percent experience bowel dysfunction. Bowel training usually begins with timed defecation (initially sometimes aided by use of glycerine suppository), increased dietary fiber in the diet, adequate liquid intake, and stool softeners if needed. Laxatives should be avoided as they may increase constipation over time. Regular use of a suppository may be indicated with persistent fecal incontinence to better control defecation.

39. A: When conducting a pelvic exam, the vaginal discharge can be evaluated with pH paper as a guide to determine whether the patient has hypoestrogenization. If the estrogen level is normal and there is no infection present, pH levels should be less than or equal to 5. An increase in pH (5.5 to 7) correlates with vaginal atrophy. A low pH serves as protection against bacterial infection, so atrophic vaginitis, which increases pH, puts the patient at increased risk of infection.

40. D: Parameters that must be set for pelvic floor electrical stimulation include amplitude, ramping, frequency rate, and duty cycle, which is the on and off rate. Generally, the most appropriate initial setting is 1:2 (for example, 5 seconds of stimulation followed by 10 seconds of rest), since this allows adequate rest to the muscle. A setting of 1:1 may be used with some patients, especially as they show progress, but 2:1 and 3:1 are not acceptable settings because time off should never be less than time on as this can lead quickly to muscle fatigue.

41. C: Pelvic floor muscle (Kegel) exercises should be done in different positions:

- Reclining exercises are done lying flat with head on a pillow and knees bent, with feet apart slightly. Knees may be supported with a pillow to prevent tightening of thigh muscles.
- Sitting exercises are done in a straight-back chair with a firm seat and with feet planted on the floor or legs stretched out and ankles crossed.

- Standing exercises are done while holding onto a surface, such as a chair or counter, for support. Knees should be bent slightly with feet about 1 foot apart. Alternately, one can lean against a counter with hips flexed.

42. B: The schedule for clean intermittent catheterization (CIC) should be based on the patient's bladder capacity in order to avoid bladder distention, which increases the risk of urinary tract infection. In this case if the patient's bladder capacity is 300 mL and the maximum output is about 1500 mL, then the patient should schedule about 5 CICs daily. Studies have indicated higher rates of infection occur with lower frequency of CIC, so a routine schedule of 5 to 6 times daily is indicated for most patients.

43. A: The initial treatment for post-prostatectomy incontinence is usually the least invasive. Since these symptoms are consistent with bladder spasms, anticholinergics may reduce spasms and incontinence with more invasive treatment done if medications are ineffective. Anticholinergics, such as Ditropan and Detrol serve to relax detrusor and pelvic floor muscles and reduce frequency. They may also increase bladder capacity and are useful for overactive bladder because they block the chemicals that stimulate bladder nerves.

44. D: Bladder capacity is assessed 3 different ways. Functional capacity is the volume of urine the bladder can hold before sensations of urgency occur. Anatomic capacity is the upper volume limit that the bladder is able to hold because of the intrinsic properties of the bladder musculature and elasticity. This is the volume when the patient is anesthetized or sedated. Cystometric capacity is the volume of urine the bladder is able to hold during urodynamic studies.

45. A: Overflow incontinence, which usually occurs with urinary retention, is most likely to occur at night when the patient is lying in supine or prone position because the bladder becomes distended during the night. Urge incontinence often occurs with increased fluid intake and triggering activities, such as hearing the sound of running water. Stress incontinence often occurs with increased activities, such as participation in sports. Mixed incontinence usually involves stress and urge incontinence, with a mixture of those symptoms.

46. A: With uroflowmetry, the normal flow pattern is usually a Bell curve with maximum or peak flow of greater than 15 mL per second. Uroflowmetry is done after the patient has a full bladder and experiences the urge to urinate. The patient urinates into a special container that measures the output in mL per second. The average volume of voided urine for adults is greater than 150 mL with residual volume of less than 100 mL acceptable in most adults.

47. B: A transducer is inserted through the urethra into the bladder and then removed at a constant rate to allow measurement of the pressures along the entire length of the urethra. Pressure may also be measured during filling of the bladder or urinating. The patient may be asked to carry out various procedures, such as coughing or carrying out the Valsalva maneuver. A special type of catheter with side holes drilled into it may also be used but with less accuracy.

48. D: For electromyography using skin surface sensors about the anus, two electrodes are used and are placed on each side of the anus at the 3 and 9 o'clock positions with a ground electrode usually placed on an inner thigh. Hair about the anus should be trimmed but not shaved (which may result in irritation), and electrodes should not be placed over scars, hemorrhoids, or irritated tissue. Skin surface sensors are indicated for those with vaginal atrophy, pregnancy, or active infection as well as when the patient is menstruating, has severe pelvic pain, or has had recent rectal or pelvic surgery.

49. C: Because the scope with instruments is passed through the urethra into the bladder, the most common adverse effect after the procedure is dysuria because trauma to the urethra causes edema, which can result in urinary retention. This is usually a transient problem, but the patient may require catheterization to empty the bladder. Infection can also occur although antibiotic prophylaxis is often giving to lessen risk of infection. Bleeding is usually mild and stops without intervention.

50. C: With the Q-tip test, a change in angle of greater than 30 degrees indicates hypermobility. The test is usually conducted with the patient lying supine and may be repeated with the patient standing. A sterile cotton swab that has been lubricated with an anesthetic jelly (such as Lidocaine) is inserted through the urethra and into the bladder and then gently pulled back until resistance is met (from the urethra). The patient bears down maximally and the angle between the stem of the cotton swab and the floor is estimated or measured with a goniometer in both resting and straining positions.

51. D: For the bowel transit time test, patients take capsules that contain radiopaque markers and then continue with their regular diet. They return 5 days later for radiographs. Typically, about 80% of the markers are excreted in 5 days, so if fewer than 20% remain, then transit time is faster than normal and more than 20%, slower than normal. This test results are affected by the types of foods and amount of liquids consumed, so results must be evaluated in terms of diet and other factors.

52. A: The rectoanal inhibitory reflex causes the internal anal sphincter to relax in response to increased rectal pressure from stool. This relaxation allows the stool to move forward and contact the proximal anal canal, which triggers sensory recognition (sampling reflex) of the contents of the rectum (formed stool, liquid stool, flatus) and the appropriate response. In patients with fecal incontinence, the rectoanal inhibitory reflex may be impaired. The ability to recognize rectal fullness may be impaired with some types of neurological diseases so that the sphincters cannot hold the increased volume.

53. B: While all of these are important factors in fecal incontinence, the most common cause is fecal impaction, which may result from chronic constipation. Chronic constipation increases pressure on the anal sphincters and can damage nerves and muscles. Additionally, transit time through the large intestine is often slowed with constipation, increasing fluid absorption and contributing to impaction. When stool becomes impacted, the body compensates by increasing fluid in the stool above the impaction, resulting in diarrhea stool leaking about the impaction and through the damaged sphincters.

54. A: The balloon expulsion test evaluates the general ability to defecate. For the test, a balloon is inserted into the rectum and filled with fluid, slowly in 10 mL increments until the patient first feels the pressure (threshold), which is usually at about 20 mL. The balloon is then filled until the patient feels an intense urge to defecate. After this, the patient sits on the toilet and attempts to expel the balloon. Normal expulsion time is about 1 minute or less, so if expulsion takes longer, this indicates some problem with coordination of muscles necessary to have a normal bowel movement.

55. C: Caffeine is a bowel irritant that may cause of increase diarrhea. Caffeine is found in coffee, tea, energy drinks, and chocolate. Other bowel irritants include cured and smoked meats, some dairy products (cheese and yogurt may decrease diarrhea), raw fruits (apples, pears, peaches, plums), fatty foods, and some artificial sweeteners (xylitol, fructose, mannitol, and sorbitol), such as those found in low calorie carbonated drinks and sugar-free gum. Alcohol may also cause diarrhea, especially in those with long-term alcohol abuse.

56. B: Waist-to-hip ratio:

Gender	Ideal	Increased risk	High risk
Male	0.9 to 0.95	0.96 to 1.0	>1.0
Female	0.7 to 0.8	0.81 to 0.85	>0.85

Measurement is done at the smallest point of the abdomen (usually above the umbilicus) and at the widest point of the hips to determine if a patient is pear-shaped (carrying fat deposits in the hips and thighs) or apple-shaped (carrying fat deposits in the abdomen). Those with apple shapes are most at risk for obesity-related health problems.

57. C: The provocative stress (cough) test requires a volume of greater than 150 mL but generally without the urge to urinate. The test is performed with the patient standing and/or lying supine. The patient is asked to cough deeply 3 times in a row. If urinary leakage occurs immediately as the patient coughs, then a presumptive diagnosis of stress incontinence is made. However, if leakage is delayed, then the patient may have other types of urinary incontinence. If a prolapse is present, it should be reduced prior to the test.

58. D: While there may be some variation depending on diagnosis, the usual preferred fluid modification for an older adult with nocturia is to increase fluid intake in the morning and afternoon to compensate for restricting fluid intake after 6 PM. Other measures to decrease nocturia include elevating legs and feet in the afternoon to reduce peripheral edema before bedtime, taking diuretics 6 hours before bedtime, eliminating caffeine drinks in the evening, and scheduled toileting around midnight.

59. B: While all of these may be included as part of teaching patients, the crucial element for bladder training is distraction and relaxation techniques since the goal is to decrease the frequency of urination by gradually extending the time between scheduled urinations (sometimes starting with every 30 minutes initially). If patients feel the urge to urinate before the scheduled time, they should use distraction or relaxation techniques and self-affirming statements to help control the urge and delay urination.

60. C: The underlying cause for obsessive toileting is usually the fear of incontinence, often for those with a neurogenic bladder. As a defense mechanism to prevent incontinence, people begin to urinate more and more frequently until they almost constantly feel the urge to urinate and may go to the toilet every few minutes. The patients undergo bladder training with scheduled toileting to increase the time between urinations. Ultrasound bladder scans are sometimes used to provide feedback to patients about bladder volume.

61. A: Posterior tibial nerve stimulation (PTNS) is sometimes used to treat urge incontinence or other urination abnormalities. This nerve contains L4-S3 nerve fibers and originates from the same nerve root that enervates the bladder. The nerve is located above the medial malleolus, and a 34-gauge needle inserted with a grounding surface electrode on the calcaneus on the same side. When the voltage is turned on, correct placement of the needle should result in the great toe bending downward. Treatments are usually one-half hour once weekly for about 3 months.

62. B: While all of these patients are at risk for functional incontinence, those at greatest risk are those who are frail and elderly because they are often dependent on others for assistance with toileting and may have physical restraints or environmental barriers that affect their ability to toilet. Functional incontinence occurs with a person is not able or not willing to use toilet facilities because of mental or physical problems although frequently functional incontinence is associated with other lower urinary tract problems, such as stress incontinence or urge incontinence.

63. D: Patients with spinal cord injury often undergo periods of spinal shock for weeks or months after injury, interfering with all reflex activity below the level of injury. This results in an atonic bladder that does not contract, even when the bladder is markedly distended, so the patient develops acute urinary retention. If the level of injury does not involve the S2-S4 segments or the cauda equina, detrusor function should resume as the spinal shock abates.

64. B: Smoking is the greatest risk factor; smokers have twice the rate of bladder cancer as nonsmokers. Carcinogens in lungs enter blood stream, are filtered by kidneys, and concentrated in urine, damaging bladder lining. Regarding race/genetics, the Caucasian rate is twice that of others. Family clusters occur. Age/Gender: More than 70% are older than 65 years. Men's rate is twice that of women. Chronic cystitis: Especially with indwelling catheters or bladders left intact after urinary diversion. Other: Exposure to aniline dye and aromatic amines and other organic chemicals, previous bladder cancer, congenital defects, chemotherapy/radiation, arsenic in drinking water, parasites, and low fluid consumption.

65. B: Creatinine clearance provides the most accurate assessment of how the kidneys will metabolize a drug. The formula for estimating creatinine clearance is:

> CC = (140 – age) X lean wt. (kg)/ 72 X serum creatinine.
> Multiply results by 0.85 for females

Because creatinine is a product of muscle breakdown and older adults have less muscle mass than younger adults, serum creatinine, which can be used to estimate creatinine clearance, is less reliable. BUN levels can be affected by multiple factors, including hydration, nutrition (especially protein intake), and muscle mass. Urinalysis cannot provide adequate information.

66. D: Extremities should be examined using modified movements that are not overly vigorous, such as pushing a limb into flexion or extension. The nurse should avoid having patients hop on one foot or do deep bends because of decreased ROM, reflexes, and balance and should always provide support of the limbs during inspection. Positioning is an issue for many older adults, who may have limited range of motion or difficulty sitting or lying in certain positions, based on their individual physical limitations. Positioning must be adjusted according to what is most comfortable for the patients, and changes of positions should be minimized.

67. A: Some sports activities may increase pressure on the bladder and increase risk of developing stress urinary incontinence, especially those activities that involve running and jumping. These include combat sports (karate, judo, jujitsu) and team sports (volleyball, basketball, handball). Other activities that increase risk are horseback riding, swinging a golf club, and heavy weightlifting. Generally, those with stress incontinence should avoid high impact sports. Low impact sports activities, such as walking, swimming, low-impact aerobics, and bicycling, pose little increased risk.

68. B: The most important factor to assess for a male considering use of a penile clamp is penile sensation because a patient with normal sensation can generally sense when the clamp is too restrictive, but if sensation is impaired, the clamp may be fastened too tightly, resulting in cyanosis and tissue damage. Clamps are most effective for those with mild urinary incontinence and should be released at least every 2 hours. Clamps are sized according to penile circumference, not length.

69. C: While there is some individual variation, the normal transit time of stool through the colon is 36 to 72 hours. The large intestine is about 1.5 meters long and comprises the cecum below the ileocecal opening and the colon (ascending, transverse, descending, and sigmoid), ending with the rectum and anal canal. The large intestine has little involvement in digestion but absorbs fluid (about 90% of the fluid that enters) and electrolytes. Stool moves through the colon through peristalsis, which occurs in the large colon only 2 to 3 times daily, usually after meals.

70. A: With an enterocele, the top or proximal portion of the vagina herniates, allowing a loop of the small intestine to prolapse through the herniated section. Pressure against the vagina occurs when the small intestine descends into the lower pelvis. Hysterectomy, childbirth, and age-related changes increase the risk of enterocele. In some cases, patients with enterocele may also have rectocele, cystocele, or uterine prolapse. Many people have no overt symptoms although some may complain of vaginal discomfort, low back pain, or dyspareunia.

71. B: Menopause is directly associated with atrophic vaginitis. This occurs as the mucoid tissues, which are estrogen-dependent, begin to thin and dry as mucoid secretions decrease. This in turn can result in irritation and can affect the urinary tract, causing urinary tract infections. Menopause, which results in weakness of the paravaginal tissues, also is associated with increased risk of cystocele, rectocele, and vaginal prolapse.

72. D: Because of the proximity of the anus to the urethra, the most common cause of a first urinary infection is *E. coli*, accounting for almost 90% of infections, with infection with *Staphylococcus aureus* accounting for 5 to 10%. Infections with other organisms, such as *Pseudomonas* are uncommon but may occur in those who are catheterized, especially with long-term continuous catheterization. Women are more at risk for urinary infections than males because of physical differences and menopausal changes.

73. A: Because of concerns about long-term use of oral estrogen, transvaginal estrogen is usually recommended for treatment of urogenital atrophy in women and may help to reduce urinary urgency and frequency. Urogenital atrophy should begin to remit within a few days to several weeks of treatment. Transvaginal estrogen reduces pH in the vagina and decreases incidence of urinary tract infections. Transvaginal estrogen is supplied as vaginal cream, vaginal tablets and a vaginal ring, which is left in place for 90 days.

74. D: The best choice for a male who occasionally dribbles small amounts of urine is probably the drip collector sock, which fits over the end of the penis and has a stretchable elastic band at the top. Most can absorb up to 2 ounces of urine and contain a plastic layer to prevent leakage. Perineal pads are usually used for females, but the leaf-shaped guard pad is similar and intended for males; but, like perineal pads, the guard attaches to underwear by an adhesives strip and doesn't work well with boxer shorts because of their loose fit.

75. C: Superabsorbent polymer (SAP) is comprised of a hydrocolloid material that changes into gel form with contact with liquid. SAP can absorb up to 70 times its weight. When placed as an inner core, it spreads the liquid throughout the product and prevents leakage although high volume products often also have a plastic outside layer because if the volume exceeds the SAP capacity, some leakage may still occur. Patients should be advised to buy products that contain SAP.

76. D: Latex and coated latex products all increase the risk of latex sensitivity and for that reason should be avoided for long-term or repeated use. The best choice for most patients is a 100% silicone catheter. Silicone catheters have wider lumens and tend to have less encrustation than other types of catheters. Teflon coating may cause irritation and encrustation because it is not completely smooth. Silicone coating is smoother but tends to dissolve over time.

77. B: The catheter insertion site (suprapubic) or meatus should be cleansed gently with soap and water or, if the patient is able, by showering. Antiseptics, such as povidone-iodine, and topical antibiotics should be avoided. Women with indwelling catheters should cleanse the perineal area after each bowel movement to prevent migration of fecal bacteria up the catheter, and men with an intact foreskin should retract the foreskin each day to cleanse the tissue of smegma, which can harbor bacteria.

78. A: Grade 1. The Baden-Walker grading scale for pelvic organ prolapse includes:

- Grade 0: No prolapse is present.
- Grade 1: Prolapse extends halfway down vagina toward the hymen.
- Grade 2: Prolapse extends entirely down the vagina to the hymen.
- Grade 3: Prolapse extends halfway down past the hymen.
- Grade 4: Prolapse of vagina, vaginal vault, and uterus extends completely outside of the hymen.

Some clinicians use a mild to severe classification with mild corresponding to grade 1, moderate to grade 2, and severe to grades 3 and 4.

79. D: Despite recent concerns about complications resulting from mesh used for some sling procedures, the midurethral sling remains the most common surgical procedure to treat stress urinary incontinence. A piece of tissue or synthetic material attaches to the pubic bone and creates a sling about the urethra. As abdominal pressure increases pressure on the bladder, the sling pulls the urethra toward the pubic bone, obstructing urine flow. Different approaches include use of tension-free vaginal tape (TVT), transobturator tape (TOT), and suprapubic arch sling (SPARC).

80. C: The most common method that women use to avoid incontinence is abstinence, avoiding sexual intimacy because of embarrassment and concerns about hygiene. However, incontinence may be reduced if women try different positions (such as the female on top, which allows better control of the pelvic muscles, or rear entry, which reduces pressure on the bladder), practice pre-coital urination, use a diaphragm (which helps prevent leakage), practice pelvic floor exercises, and place absorbent pads on the bed. Urine leakage during sexual activity is more common with females because the engorged penis blocks urine flow in the male urethra.

81. D: If teaching a patient with spinal cord injury to do digital stimulation, the patient should be advised that once the rectum starts to empty, the patient should place the finger on one side and continue the stimulation during the entire defecation and for 5 additional minutes to ensure that all stool has been expelled. The patient should stimulate the rectum and attempt to promote evacuation for at least 20 minutes before stopping. Digital stimulation may also be done with a special device called a dill stick.

82. A: If a patient has recently developed intermittent fecal incontinence, the first step in developing patient-centered goals is to assess the patient's normal defecation pattern over the preceding weeks to determine what variables may be evident. Maintaining a bowel diary for 3 to 7 days may also be very helpful because patients are not always accurate reporters. Any causative factors should be identified, such as changes in medications, activity, or foods, that may be contributing to the incontinence.

83. C: If a patient is undergoing bowel training in the morning after breakfast with a bisacodyl suppository, digital stimulation be carried out every 10 to 15 minutes after the suppository is inserted until evacuation. If digital stimulation is done too soon, it may cause the suppository to be expelled so an adequate duration of time must pass to give the suppository enough time to begin to stimulate contractions. If the suppository is ineffective, the patient should be assessed for fecal impaction.

84. B: If a patient has a disposable urethral insert (FemSoft®) and has inserted it with a stylus in place, the patient should remove the insert by pulling it gently straight outward. The balloon that holds the urethral insert in place is small and flattens easily when pressure is applied as it slides into the urethra. Once removed, the urethral insert is discarded. Urethral inserts may increase the risk of infection and may cause irritation of the bladder or urethra but are generally well-tolerated.

85. B: For a male patient to safely use a penile compression device, such as a pencil clamp, the patient must have normal sensation so that the patient can feel discomfort in the penis if the clamp is applied to tightly and can feel when the bladder is full. The clamp should be released for urination every hour or two because prolonged use without release may result in damage to the tissues. Various types of penile compression devices are available. One type, for example, is an inflatable ring that circles the penis. Most types of penile compression devices are reusable but should be kept clean.

86. A: If a patient has developed urinary incontinence but it's unclear if it is a transient problem, the first step should be to keep a 3-day bladder/bowel record to help to determine if there are any patterns that emerge. The bladder diary should include not only the frequency and amount of urinations but also the frequency and amount of fluid intake. A bowel record should be maintained along with the bladder record because sometimes bowel problems (such as constipation) may contribute to urinary incontinence.

87. D: Biofeedback with a pressure-sensitive probe inserted into the rectum is likely to be most effective for fecal incontinence associated with weak sphincter muscles. If the patient has weak sphincter sensation, biofeedback may be of some benefit, but not if the sensation is absent. Those with underlying neurological disease usually see little benefit from biofeedback because of the nerve damage.

88. C: Holding breath may indicate recruitment of additional muscle groups when assessing a patient trying to contract pelvic floor muscles during pelvic floor muscle training. The nurse should observe the patient closely as the patient attempts to tighten the pelvic floor muscles to determine if the patient is tensing other muscles (abdomen, arms, legs), lifting heels off of the floor, curling toes under, or rising slightly off of the chair (if seated) or table (if supine).

89. A: A poorly-controlled diabetic patient has had frequent fecal impactions with overflow fecal incontinence because of chronic constipation that results from the kidneys drawing water as a solvent for unmetabolized sugar. This, in turn, results in polyuria and increases risk of dehydration and constipation if fluid intake is not adequate to compensate. Stool is from 70% to 80% water, and if it falls below that, the stool becomes hard and can easily impact.

90. C: When teaching a male patient to use a reusable external condom catheter, the nurse should advise the patient to remove the external catheter for cleaning every 24 hours. The skin should be carefully examined for signs of irritation and thoroughly washed and dried before the clean external catheter is reapplied. Different types of external catheters are available. Some secure with adhesive and others with an inflatable retention ring.

91. D: If an indwelling urinary catheter has been in place for 2 weeks and the patient's urine is cloudy, in order to obtain a urine specimen for culture and sensitivities the nurse should change the catheter and collect a specimen directly from the new catheter. Bacteria rapidly colonize urinary catheters and biofilms have formed in almost 100% by one month; so, if the catheter is not changed, the urine specimen will be contaminated with bacteria from the catheter and may not reflect what is in the urine.

92. D: The most appropriate management product for a nonambulatory patient with dementia with moderate to heavy urinary incontinence is adjustable disposable incontinence briefs with Velcro openings. This type of underwear is easiest to put on a patient who is wheelchair and bedbound. Indwelling catheters should be avoided because they invariably lead to chronic urinary infections. Incontinence briefs wick the urine away from the skin and decrease incidence of IASD.

93. A: The type of diagnostic study that is most effective in diagnosing the type of urinary incontinence a patient is experiencing is the videourodynamic studies. Videourodynamic studies may include post-void residual, uroflowmetry, multichannel cystometry, urethral pressure profilometry, and fluoroscopy. Typically for the test, a catheter is inserted into the bladder and sometimes the rectum and fluid instilled and then various measurements are carried out with the bladder full and during urination.

94. B: Pessaries are most likely to become dislodged during urination and defecation because of the bearing down activity. Therefore, when fitting a pessary, it's important that the patient go through various activities, such as walking and bending, for about an hour after the pessary is inserted and then urinate to ensure that the pessary stays in place and poses no discomfort to the patient. Pessaries should not cause pain, and women, especially those who have used tampons, generally tolerate the pessary well.

95. D: Grapefruit may increase the adverse effects of oxybutynin, so patients should be advised to avoid eating grapefruit or drinking grapefruit juice. Oxybutynin is an anticholinergic/antimuscarinic drug that treats overactive bladder by relaxing the bladder muscles, reducing urge incontinence. Oxybutynin should not be used with patients with glaucoma, and patients should be cautioned to avoid high heat or exertion during hot weather because oxybutynin reduces the ability to perspire. Oxybutynin may cause blurred vision, so some patients may have to restrict driving.

96. C: If a 64-year-old female patient has persistent overflow incontinence resulting from an areflexic detrusor muscle, the recommended treatment is clean intermittent catheterization if the patient is able to carry out the procedure. A Foley catheter may be inserted but increases the risk of infection because colonization of bacteria usually occurs within 14 days. A Foley catheter should be routinely changed at least once monthly as encrustations may cause blockage and bladder spasms.

97. C: The most important factor in determining whether an event is a stressor to a patient is the patient's perception. For example, if two patients have kidneys removed for cancer and both are stage I, one patient may be relieved that the stage is low and feel very positive about recovery while the second patient may be overwhelmed with anxiety and fear at the thought of any cancer and may obsess over the possibility of recurrence.

98. A: If a woman with an overactive bladder is concerned about leaking urine during sexual intercourse and has avoided sexual intimacy, the best advice is to take steps to minimize leakage:

- Urinate immediately before intercourse.
- Place protective materials (towel, underpads) on furniture/bed.
- Limit fluids for a few hours before intercourse (but avoid dehydration).
- Try different positions during intercourse as some may put less pressure on the bladder.

99. D: If a patient is undergoing the stage one trial period with the InterStim® sacral nerve stimulator, a successful response is >50% decrease in leaking episodes per day, severity of leaking, number of absorbant products used, volume and number of voids per day, degree of urgency, number of catheterizations. Additionally, the patient should exhibit a 50% increase in voided volumes. The InterStim® provides electrical impulses to stimulate sacral nerve roots that affect urination.

100. C: The most effective position for active listening is sitting directly in front of the patient with arms and legs uncrossed so that the health nurse appears open to the patient's comments. The nurse should lean slightly toward the patient to indicate interest and should establish eye contact although the eye contact should not be overly aggressive or staring as this may be intimidating. The nurse should relax and appear comfortable with the patient.

101. D: A nonverbal clue that a patient may be anxious is if the patient rubs the hands together constantly as this is a self-comforting measure. Nonverbal behavior can include the tone of voice and cadence of speech, body positioning or behaviors (arms crossed, sitting forward, leaning backward), facial expressions (frowning, grimacing, relaxed), eye cast, amount of eye contact, obvious autonomic physiological responses (diaphoresis and blushing), personal appearance (grooming, hygiene), and physical characteristics (extreme over- or under-weight).

102. B: Medicaid in most states covers the cost of incontinent supplies, but Medicare does not. Only some private insurances cover the cost of these supplies. While some manufacturers have patient assistance programs for diabetic supplies and ostomy supplies, there are few available for incontinent supplies. Medicare, Medicaid, and private insurances generally cover the costs of catheters for those who carry out intermittent catheterization, but they may limit the number of catheters.

103. B: If a female patient with urinary incontinence reports that she feels less physically attractive and more dissatisfied with her body and finds it difficult to look at herself naked although other aspects of her life are good, this suggests an impaired body image. A negative body image is common in patients with incontinence, regardless of age. Patients often begin to feel self-conscious, worrying that people will know about the incontinence or smell urine.

104. A: If the nurse hears a patient's physician complaining that a patient is "difficult and impatient," and the nurse tells the physician that the patient is very frightened and acting defensively, the aspect of care that the nurse is exhibiting is advocacy. The nurse is speaking up in defense of the patient and acting for the patient's benefit in trying to help the physician have a more balanced view of the patient's behavior.

105. C: If a female patient is scheduled for a sling procedure to correct stress incontinence, the patient should be advised to avoid sexual intercourse for at least 6 weeks to allow time for adequate healing of the tissue. Some patients may find that sexual intercourse is painful when intimate relations resume. Patients should also avoid strenuous exercise and heavy lifting for the first 2 to 4 weeks. Sling procedures are often done as outpatient procedures and are well-tolerated by most patients.

106. B: When applying no-sting barrier film (such as Cavilon™ spray) to protect the skin from urinary or fecal incontinence, the spay container should be held 4 to 6 inches above the skin. One area should be sprayed and then another area rather than spraying back and forth over the same area. The film should be allowed to dry thoroughly. In some cases, a second layer may be applied after the first layer has dried to provide a greater barrier.

107. C: Soap and water are the least effective in protecting the skin from incontinence-associated dermatitis because the soap tends to dry the skin, making it more vulnerable to the effects of urine and stool. Products that provide moisturizing as well as a skin barrier are the most effective. These products may include barrier films (which may be sprayed or painted on the skin), zinc oxide cream, petrolatum jelly, and lanolin preparations.

108. D: If a patient has developed low anterior resection syndrome with persistent fecal incontinence of semi-solid stool, Kegel exercises and dietary modifications may help to reduce the incontinence. Since the stools are semi-solid, diarrhea does not appear to be a factor, so strengthening the sphincter muscles through Kegel exercises may help. Reducing foods high in gas producing may also help to reduce incontinence. Symptoms that persist for a year or more after surgery are often permanent.

109. B: If an older adult has sudden onset of confusion, urinary incontinence, and slight unsteadiness but exhibits no focal weakness or complaints of dysuria, the nurse should suspect urinary tract infection. Older adults often present with atypical signs and symptoms of UTI because their immune system is often impaired, and marked confusion, hallucinations, and changes in behavior common. Patients are often thought to have dementia, but the symptoms clear when the UTI infection is treated.

110. A: Obesity is a risk factor for development of a cystocele. Other risk factors include pregnancy, childbirth, older age, history of hysterectomy, and genetic predisposition to weak connective tissue. A cystocele occurs when the anterior vaginal wall descends or prolapses and the muscles weaken, allowing the bladder to press into the vagina. A cystocele may press against the urethra, resulting in difficulty urinating and urinary incontinence.

111. C: Spicy foods should be avoided by those with overactive bladders because they may increase irritation of the bladder and stimulate further contractions. Other foods that may increase symptoms include carbonated, caffeinated, and alcoholic beverages; sports drinks, citrus fruits, tomatoes and tomato products, sugar substitutes, sugar, honey, chocolate, and raw onions. Patients may be more sensitive to some of these foods than others so they should be encouraged to add them one at a time to the diet to assess their response.

112. D: OnabotulinumtoxinA (Botox®) has been approved by the FDA for treatment of overactive bladder for those who have been unresponsive to anticholinergic/antimuscarinic drugs or cannot tolerate the drugs. OnabotulinumtoxinA was previously approved for urinary incontinence associated with neurological disorders (such as MS) and spinal cord injury. The medication (100 units) is injected into 10 to 20 sites in the detrusor muscle during cystoscopy. The effects wear off within about 6 months, and the procedure needs to be repeated.

113. B: A Gehrung pessary or cube pessary may be utilized for treatment of a mild rectocele. A rectocele occurs when the anterior wall of the rectum prolapses into the posterior wall of the vagina (the rectovaginal septum). Small rectoceles are often asymptomatic, but larger rectoceles may result in complications, such as pain during intercourse and bowel obstruction. Risk factors include pregnancy and childbirth as well as older age.

114. A: If a patient with overactive bladder reports that she has severely limited fluids in order to decrease incontinence, the nurse should advise the patient that this may increase bladder irritation, which in turn can increase urinary incontinence. Additionally, restricting fluids may increase the risk of infection and constipation. When cautioning a patient, the nurse should always be specific about the problems that may arise rather than making vague statements such as "serious adverse effects."

115. D: When assessing vaginal pH during a pelvic exam, the vaginal pH that is consistent with atrophic vaginitis is 5.5 to 7. The normal vaginal pH is less than 5 if the patient has adequate estrogen and no signs of infection. The normal vaginal flora includes lactobacilli, which produce substances that maintain a low pH in which most bacteria cannot thrive. However, if the number of lactobacilli decreases, an alkaline environment that encourages growth of other bacteria and atrophic changes in the vagina occurs.

116. C: Checking. The 5 steps to prompted voiding include:

1. Checking: Check the patient's clothing, linens, and absorbant protective materials on a regular schedule, allowing the patient to ask for toileting if the patient desires.
2. Talking: Ask the patient is the patient is wet or dry and verify to determine the patient's level of awareness.
3. Prompting: Prompt (at least 3 times if the patient refuses) the patient to urinate and offer to assist.
4. Praising: Provide positive feedback for staying try and using or trying to use the toilet to urinate.
5. Correcting: Remind the patient that the goal is to stay dry if the patient is incontinent.

117. D: If a patient with venous insufficiency tends to develop peripheral edema by evening and this corresponds with nocturia, the patient should be advised to wear compression stockings and elevate feet/legs in the afternoon and evening to promote circulation and movement of extravascular fluids back into the bloodstream before bedtime. If patients restrict fluids to control nocturia, they should do so only in the evening but should compensate by drinking more during earlier hours of the day so that total fluid intake is adequate.

118. A: Ulcerative proctitis is a condition that is commonly associated with tenesmus and fecal urgency. Ulcerative proctitis is a milder form of ulcerative colitis that involves primarily the rectum but may extend 20 cm into the colon. About a third to a half of those with ulcerative proctitis will progress to ulcerative colitis over time with the ulcerative lesions involving the sigmoid colon. Treatment may include dietary modification and lifestyle changes as well as antidiarrheal medications (loperamide). bulk formers (Metamucil®), and anti-inflammatory medications (5-ASA, corticosteroids.

119. C: With the Q-tip urethral test, the angle of the Q-tip with straining or coughing that corresponds to urethral hypermobility is ≥30 degrees. The Q-tip test is sometimes done to assess stress urinary incontinence in females because urethral hypermobility indicates inadequate urethra support, so pelvic floor muscle training may be helpful. If the angle is less than 30 degrees, this is consistent with intrinsic dysfunction of the urethral sphincter, and pelvic floor muscle training is likely to be ineffective.

120. A: If utilizing double voiding for urinary retention, the patient should urinate and then remain seated and urinate again in 2 to 10 minutes. The duration of time should be individualized for the patient to determine which duration tends to be most effective. Some patients may find it more effective to urinate, stand up, and then sit down and urinate again. Double voiding is generally not effective if urinary retention is severe.

Practice Test #2

1. Which of the following medications may be administered for detrusor underactivity?

a. Duloxetine
b. Oxybutynin
c. Imipramine
d. Bethanechol

2. The drainage bag of an indwelling catheter should be emptied at least every

a. 2 hours.
b. 4 to 6 hours.
c. 8 hours.
d. 12 hours.

3. What is the most common self-care method both males and females use to manage urinary incontinence?

a. remaining homebound
b. defensive urination
c. toilet mapping
d. limiting fluid intake

4. What is usually the first step in treating a fecal impaction?

a. administer an oil retention enema
b. do manual removal
c. administer a laxative
d. administer a stimulant suppository

5. On pelvic exam of a patient with vaginal itching, soreness, burning, and dyspareunia, the nurse notes a small amount of blood-tinged mucoid discharge; atrophic vulva; and dry, pale, ecchymotic vaginal mucosa. This is most consistent with a diagnosis of

a. candida vaginitis.
b. trichomonas vaginitis.
c. atrophic vaginitis.
d. bacterial vaginosis.

6. Rectosigmoidal outlet delay constipation often responds well to

a. hypnosis.
b. biofeedback.
c. laxatives and stool softeners.
d. increased fiber in diet.

7. Patients who have chronic constipation and must strain to defecate have increased risk of

a. urinary tract infections.
b. migraines.
c. upper GI bleeding.
d. cholecystitis.

8. During the initial trial period for prompted voiding, the first intervention is to

a. schedule verbal reminders and provide positive feedback.
b. ask patients if they want to use the toilet.
c. modify fluid intake.
d. ask patients if they are wet or dry, check, and provide feedback.

9. Using the Urinary Incontinence Severity Index, a patient who experiences incontinence a few times a week in small splashes would be classified as

a. slight.
b. moderate.
c. severe.
d. very severe.

10. What is the primary risk factor for fecal incontinence?

a. vaginal delivery
b. institutionalization of the elderly
c. chronic disease
d. anorectal surgery

11. Which of the following is a risk factor for urge incontinence?

a. obesity
b. vaginal delivery
c. chronic cough
d. stroke

12. Which of the following is an example of a problem with emptying of the bladder?

a. acute and chronic urinary retention
b. neurogenic dysfunction (reflex incontinence)
c. stress incontinence
d. functional incontinence

13. The bladder of an adult can usually hold

a. 200 to 400 mL.
b. 300 to 600 mL.
c. 600 to 800 mL.
d. 800 to 1000 mL.

14. In older adult females, the nurse should expect

a. increased stress urinary incontinence.
b. decreased urge incontinence.
c. decreased stress incontinence and increased urge incontinence.
d. increased stress and urge incontinence.

15. Which type of pelvic organ prolapse is most likely to result in fecal incontinence?

a. enterocele
b. rectocele
c. cystocele
d. rectal prolapse

16. What is the longest duration that a pessary should be left in place?

a. 6 weeks
b. 2 years
c. 12 months
d. 4 months

17. Which of the following treatments is most indicated for a frail 82-year-old female who has developed second-degree uterovaginal prolapse?

a. Hodge pessary
b. donut pessary
c. ring pessary
d. referral to surgeon for surgical repair

18. What is the best advice to a caregiver of a 72-year-old male with dementia of the Alzheimer type who has been getting up between midnight and 2 AM to urinate, but gets confused and urinates on the floor?

a. restrict patient's fluids in the evening
b. place Depends or other disposable undergarments on the patient at bedtime
c. provide patient with a bedside urinal
d. get patient up for scheduled toileting at midnight

19. When assessing an elderly patient's functional ability, which test is used specifically to indicate risk of falls?

a. timed up and go (TUG)
b. Katz Activities of Daily Living Scale
c. Functional Ability Rating Scale
d. Instrumental Activities of Daily Living

20. When fitting a penile sheath to a 76-year-old male with persistent dribbling of urine, which measurement is most important?

a. retracted penile length
b. erect penile length
c. flaccid penile length
d. penile circumference

21. Scattered 0.2 to 0.5 cm serous fluid-filled skin lesions would be described as

a. macules.
b. papules.
c. vesicles.
d. bullas.

22. A female patient with ectopia of the ureter (vaginal) would likely experience

a. vaginal leakage of urine.
b. urinary retention.
c. vaginitis.
d. vaginismus.

23. Urination by classic reflex mechanism occurs with

a. older adults.
b. toddlers.
c. adults.
d. infants.

24. In male patients, which of the following is the most significant factor in change in male urinary sphincter function?

a. prostatic cancer
b. benign prostatic hypertrophy
c. bladder cancer
d. rectal cancer

25. On scrotal examination, the nurse feels a soft mass but can get the examining finger above the mass, which transilluminates on further examination, suggesting the mass is a(n)

a. epidermoid cyst.
b. varicocele.
c. hydrocele.
d. scrotal hernia.

26. The normal length of the prostate gland palpated on rectal exam is about

a. 1 to 2 cm.
b. 2.5 cm.
c. 3.5 to 4 cm.
d. 4 to 5 cm.

27. What is the best schedule for changing indwelling catheters?

a. as needed
b. weekly
c. bi-weekly
d. monthly

28. What is the best time to take a loop diuretic (such as furosemide) to reduce nocturia?

a. early morning
b. bedtime
c. noon
d. 6 hours before bedtime

29. Hesitancy related to urination refers to

a. starting and stopping of urine flow.
b. reduced force of urine flow.
c. difficulty starting urine flow and delayed onset.
d. the need to use intra-abdominal pressure to increase urine flow.

30. What is the primary obstacle to patient's receiving treatment for incontinence?

a. patient's embarrassment
b. lack of information
c. health giver's reluctant to discuss the issue
d. lack of access to care

31. In a bowel diary, the Bristol Stool Form Scale is used to

a. describe the frequency of incontinence.
b. differentiate between defecation and incontinence.
c. describe the amount of stool.
d. describe the type of stool.

32. Contained incontinence means that the patient

a. is only incontinent in some circumstances.
b. must use absorbent products to contain urinary leakage.
c. controls incontinence with scheduled toileting.
d. controls incontinence with medications.

33. A patient with multiple sclerosis who has persistent severe urinary retention because of inability to relax the sphincters is most likely treated with

a. catheterization with continuous drainage.
b. oxybutynin.
c. clean intermittent catheterization.
d. baclofen.

34. Which of the following control methods is most appropriate for a 45-year-old woman who states that she sometimes leaks a small amount of urine when she coughs or sneezes?

a. using a urethral plug
b. taking an anticholinergic agent daily
c. wearing protective incontinence pads
d. using the "knack" to prevent incontinence

35. Which of the following is probably the best use of a urethral insert to control stress incontinence?

a. use during specific time periods, such as during working hours
b. use during specific activities, such as playing tennis
c. routine nighttime use
d. routine daytime use

36. Vaginal weights are most effective as part of the treatment regimen for which of the following types of incontinence?

a. functional incontinence
b. urge incontinence
c. stress incontinence
d. mixed urinary incontinence

37. If, when conducting a digital pelvic exam with evaluation of the pelvic floor muscles, the nurse feels no compression of the muscles, what should be the next step?

a. press on the posterior vaginal wall
b. press on the anterior vaginal wall
c. remove the fingers and reinsert
d. terminate digital examination

38. Which of the following treatments is most likely to be effective for a patient with intrinsic urethral sphincter dysfunction (ISD)?

a. periurethral injection
b. pelvic floor muscle exercises
c. pessary
d. electrical stimulation

39. When setting the amplitude for pelvic floor electrical stimulation, what finding indicates adequate electrical current?

a. patient reports vibration
b. anal wink occurs with stimulation
c. patient reports urge to urinate during stimulation
d. slight pain with contraction of pelvic floor muscle

40. What is the most effective treatment for a patient with an indwelling catheter and a urine pH of 5.6?

a. cranberry tablets, 400 mg BID
b. no treatment indicated
c. cranberry juice, 2 glasses daily
d. ascorbic acid, 1 g daily

41. Which of the following techniques is the easiest method for a patient to check if the pelvic floor muscles are flexing when a patient is learning to do pelvic floor muscle (Kegel) exercises?

a. stop flow of urine in midst of urination
b. pull in the anus as though trying to stop from passing flatus
c. lie supine, place finger inside vagina and squeeze as though trying to stop urine
d. hold breath while trying to pull in anus as though stopping flatus

42. With a 260 mL volume of voided urine, the residual volume of an adult patient is expected to be less than

a. 30 mL.
b. 60 mL.
c. 100 mL.
d. 200 mL.

43. Which surgical procedure is probably the most effective for treatment of severe post-prostatectomy incontinence?

a. insertion of artificial sphincter
b. injection of bulking agent about urethra
c. sacral nerve stimulation
d. urethral sling procedure

44. Patients with diabetic neuropathy are most at risk for which of the following types of incontinence?

a. stress urinary incontinence
b. overflow urinary incontinence
c. mixed urinary incontinence
d. functional incontinence

45. Which of the following drugs is most likely to be effective for a 64-year-old female who has developed chronic urge incontinence because of an overactive bladder?

a. Oxybutynin
b. Sertraline
d. Duloxetine
c. Desmopressin

46. When teaching a female patient to do clean intermittent catheterization (CIC), how far should the nurse instruct the patient to initially insert the catheter?

a. 1 to 2 inches
b. 2 to 3 inches
c. 3 to 4 inches
d. 4 to 5 inches

47. Which of the following diagnostic procedures includes inflation of a balloon into the rectum to assess anal sphincter function and neural reflexes?

a. anal sphincter electromyography
b. endoanal ultrasound
c. anal manometry
d. pudendal nerve terminal motor latency test

48. Using the PLISSIT model for assessing sexuality, which of the following should the nurse do first when speaking to a patient?

a. ask permission to discuss sexual function
b. provide limited information about sexual function
c. provide suggestions for dealing with erectile dysfunction
d. suggest intensive therapy

49. With uroflowmetry, an explosive flow pattern with a steeper than normal pattern but a shorter urinating time most likely indicates

a. deficient detrusor function.
b. bladder outlet obstruction.
c. mixed incontinence.
d. stress incontinence.

50. During cystometry, maximum cystometric capacity is reached when the patient

a. first feels bladder pressure.
b. has strong urge to urinate and cannot delay.
c. feels the need to urinate but is able to delay.
d. feels a persistent need to urinate but is not afraid of leakage.

51. What is the purpose of conducting urodynamic testing for abdominal leak point pressure (ALPP)?

a. determine the strength of the pelvic floor muscles
b. measure detrusor contraction
c. determine urethral sphincter competence
d. determine bladder outlet obstruction

52. Which type of sedation is usually indicated for flexible sigmoidoscopy?

a. minimal
b. moderate/conscious sedation
c. deep sedation
d. general anesthesia

53. Which next treatment is most appropriate for a 56-year-old female with a normal colonoscopy but frequent constipation despite taking occasional laxatives or water enemas to prevent impaction and increasing fiber and fluids in diet?

a. daily stool softener, such as Colace
b. daily bulk former, such as Metamucil
c. small daily dose of laxative, such as Milk of Magnesia
d. routine saline enemas

54. Which test is most likely indicated for a patient with suspected tearing or scar tissue of the anal sphincters?

a. MRI
b. anal electromyography
c. endoanal ultrasonography
d. balloon expulsion test

55. Which of the following older adult patients should probably avoid a high-fiber diet to control constipation?

a. a patient with impaired rectal sensation
b. a patient with impaired sphincter function
c. a patient with hypomotility and reduced bowel transit time
d. a patient with hypermotility and increased bowel transit time

56. The KUB (kidney, ureters, and bladder) x-ray may aid in the diagnosis of

a. detrusor sphincter dyssynergia.
b. stress incontinence.
c. urinary retention.
d. constipation and kidney stones.

57. Oxybutynin TDS should be applied to the skin how often?

a. daily
b. 2 times weekly
c. 3 times weekly
d. every 2 weeks

58. Patients scheduled for a renal and bladder ultrasound must be advised

a. to urinate prior to the ultrasound.
b. to fast for 12 hours except for water.
c. that no preparation is necessary.
d. to ensure a full bladder for the ultrasound.

59. Which of the following waist measurements for a female is considered a risk factor for obesity-related health conditions?

a. less than or equal to 35 inches
b. greater than 35 inches
c. 36 to 40 inches
d. greater than 40 inches

60. When conducting a one-hour pad test, the patient is asked to

a. bring wet incontinence pads to the office for evaluation.
b. carry out provocative activities.
c. carry out normal activities, such as walking.
d. refrain from drinking for 4 hours before the test.

61. When assessing the urethral pressure profile (UPP) during urodynamic studies, the urethral closure pressure is calculated by

a. subtracting the intravesical pressure from the intraurethral pressure.
b. adding the intravesical pressure and the intraurethral pressure.
c. multiplying the intravesical pressure by the intraurethral pressure.
d. dividing the intravesical pressure by the intraurethral pressure.

62. When treating transient urinary incontinence, the first step is to

a. restrict fluids.
b. change medications.
c. determine cause.
d. prevent constipation.

63. What is the total recommended daily fluid intake (from foods and fluids) for an adult male?

a. 1.5 L
b. 2.7 L
c. 3 L
d. 3.7 L

64. When teaching a patient to double void to help control urinary retention, how much rest period should usually elapse between urinations?

a. 30 to 60 seconds
b. 1 to 2 minutes
c. 2 to 10 minutes
d. 15 to 20 minutes

65. Smoking is most associated with which type of incontinence?

a. stress
b. overflow
c. urge
d. reflex

66. In order to reduce stress incontinence by about 50%, what percentage of weight loss should a morbidly obese patient target?

a. 2 to 5%
b. 5 to 10%
c. 10 to 15%
d. 15 to 20%

67. What is the best response to a patient who is undergoing habit training for urination and feels the need to urinate prior to the scheduled toileting time?

a. allow the patient to urinate
b. insist the patient delay urination
c. encourage the patient to urinate whenever he or she feels the urge
d. ask the patient to delay urination unless the urge is unbearable

68. Which of the following assessment tools is most indicated for a 76-year-old male recovering from prostatectomy exhibiting sudden onset of confusion with fluctuating inattention, disorganized thinking, and altered level of consciousness?

a. Mini-mental state exam (MMSE)
b. Mini-Cog
c. Confusion assessment method (CAM)
d. Geriatric depression scale (GDS)

69. Which age-related change to the gastrointestinal system is most likely to result in constipation?

a. smooth muscle in colon is less responsive to neural stimulation
b. intestinal walls thin
c. chyme exits the stomach more slowly
d. rectal walls are less elastic

70. Which type of incontinence is most likely to cause a person to leak urine at the sound of running water?

a. stress
b. overflow
c. urge
d. functional

71. What is the most likely cause of a urine culture report indicating multiple organisms?

a. poor patient hygiene
b. specimen contamination
c. immunosuppression
d. chronic infection

72. What is the most likely cause of a 42-year-old woman reporting her menstrual cycle length is becoming shorter?

a. uterine cancer
b. pelvic inflammatory disease
c. vaginitis
d. perimenopause

73. What is the most common side effect of antimuscarinic drugs for treatment of overactive bladder?

a. drowsiness
b. dizziness
c. blurred vision
d. dry mouth

74. Which of the following absorbent products is the best choice for a bedridden patient incontinent of large amounts of urine and feces?

a. mesh pants with disposable inserts
b. disposable underpads
c. reusable protective underwear
d. disposable adult diaper-like brief

75. Which of the following is the best choice for a skin barrier for a patient with perineal dermatitis from frequent exposure to liquid stool?

a. zinc oxide
b. petrolatum
c. lanolin
d. dimethicone

76. When botulinum toxin A (BTX-A) is used for bladder overactivity, how many injections are usually made into the bladder wall?

a. 5 to 10
b. 10 to 20
c. 20 to 30
d. 30 to 40

77. The bran-containing recipe for treatment of chronic constipation also includes

a. bananas and yogurt.
b. prune juice and yogurt.
c. raw apples and prune juice.
d. applesauce and prune juice.

78. What is the most common complication resulting from long-term catheter use?

a. catheter-associated urinary infection
b. urethral trauma
c. hematuria
d. bladder stones

79. In normal urination, the first sensation of the need to urinate should occur when the bladder is about

a. one-quarter full.
b. one-half full.
c. three-quarters full.
d. full.

80. Which ethnic group of females has the highest prevalence of stress urinary incontinence?

a. Hispanics
b. African Americans
c. Asians
d. Caucasians

81. If using vaginal weights as part of pelvic floor muscle training, the weights should be held in place for

a. up to 60 minutes BID.
b. up to 45 minutes BID.
c. up to 30 minutes BID.
d. up to 15 minutes BID.

82. When educating a patient about medications, the nurse should advise the patient that the most common adverse effect of anticholinergic/antimuscarinic drugs is

a. tachycardia and cardiac irregularities.
b. insomnia.
c. dry mouth and constipation.
d. orthostatic hypotension.

83. If an older male patient has been using curved leaf incontinent pads for mild urinary incontinence but complains that they won't stay in place and sometimes fall out, the nurse should ask the patient,

a. "What style of underwear do you wear?"
b. "Have you tried a larger size?"
c. "Would you like to try pull-ons"
d. "Have you considered using a condom catheter?"

84. Which type of support group for patients with fecal incontinence is likely to be the most acceptable to the majority of patients who are referred?

a. non-specific
b. gender specific
c. age specific
d. cause specific

85. Which of a patient's medications may be contributing to fecal incontinence?

a. metformin
b. levothyroxine
c. metoprolol
d. vitamin D

86. Which of the following is a contraindication to the use of a fecal pouch?

a. patient is non-ambulatory
b. stool is formed
c. patient is ambulatory
d. patient needs assistance to reposition

87. Which of the following forms a lipid barrier to protect skin against loss of water?

a. emollient
b. humectant
c. hydrating agent
d. anti-inflammatory agent

88. If a patient has involuntary loss of flatus, mucus, and feces without sensation or urge, this type of incontinence is classified as

a. functional fecal incontinence.
b. passive fecal incontinence.
c. functional flatus incontinence.
d. passive anal incontinence.

89. When beginning percutaneous tibial nerve stimulation and adjusting the setting, if the great toe dorsiflexes at a setting of 12, what setting should be used for the treatment?

a. 10
b. 11
c. 12
d. 13

90. If a patient has an artificial anal sphincter and deflates the balloon to have a bowel movement, the sphincter will automatically refill after

a. 20 minutes.
b. 15 minutes.
c. 10 minutes.
d. 5 minutes.

91. If, following a stroke, a patient has some residual paralysis and has difficulty cooking foods, engaging in recreational activities, dressing, and toileting independently, the referral that is most indicated is

a. occupational therapy.
b. physical therapy.
c. nutritionist.
d. recreational therapist.

92. If a patient is incontinent of stool only when the stool is loose, the primarily intervention is

a. absorbant pads.
b. bulking agent.
c. loperamide (Imodium®).
d. pelvic floor exercises (Kegel).

93. Following injections of a tissue bulking agent (Solesta®) to control fecal incontinence, the patient should be advised to avoid

a. mild exercise for one week.
b. solid foods for 24 hours.
c. dairy products for 3 days.
d. hot baths for 24 hours.

94. Following prostatectomy, especially radical prostatectomy, male patients may experience urinary incontinence because

a. sensation is decreased.
b. swelling impairs functioning.
c. the internal bladder neck sphincter is damaged or removed.
d. the external sphincter is damaged or removed.

95. Which of the following neurological disorders is associated with especially high rates of fecal incontinence?

a. multiple sclerosis
b. Parkinson's disease
c. cerebral palsy
d. epilepsy

96. If, during the physical examination, the patient does not exhibit the anal wink, this indicates the need for

a. sigmoidoscopy.
b. neurological examination.
c. electrolyte laboratory studies.
d. colonoscopy.

97. The volume of urine that the bladder is physically able to contain is referred to as the

a. anatomic capacity.
b. functional capacity.
c. residual capacity.
d. cytometric capacity.

98. The primary treatment for sensory urinary urgency is

a. anticholinergic/antimuscarinic.
b. surgical intervention.
c. pelvic floor electrical stimulation.
d. behavior modification.

99. When assessing the patient's bladder diary, the first thing that the nurse should verify is

a. the patient's voiding intervals.
b. the number of voidings in 24 hours.
c. the patient's pattern of waking and sleeping.
d. the pattern of urinary incontinence.

100. An absent bulbocavernosus response in a male patient is generally indicative of

a. overactive bladder.
b. denervation of spinal cord roots.
c. benign prostatic hyperplasia.
d. prostatitis.

101. Voiding intervals during waking hours should be at least

a. one hour.
b. two hours.
c. three hours.
d. four hours.

102. The initial treatment of choice for children with nocturnal enuresis is

a. desmopressin.
b. imipramine.
c. fluoxetine.
d. enuresis alarm.

103. The most common reason for failure and ultimate removal of an artificial urinary sphincter is

a. infection and/or erosion.
b. hemorrhage/hematoma.
c. rejection.
d. obstruction.

104. Hirschsprung disease should be suspected if a neonate fails to pass meconium within

a. 12 hours.
b. 24 hours.
c. 36 hours.
d. 48 hours.

105. If, despite advice to stop smoking to help control overactive bladder, a patient continues to smoke heavily, the nurse should

a. remain supportive but express concern.
b. address the behavior and offer resources.
c. say nothing out of respect for patient's rights.
d. criticize the patient's behavior and point out problems.

106. If a male newborn has hypospadias, the two other most common anomalies that are often found in association with hypospadias include

a. undescended testicles and bladder extrophy.
b. testicular torsion and inguinal hernia.
c. inguinal hernia and undescended testicles
d. ambiguous genitalia and umbilical hernia.

107. If, when reviewing a patient's food diary to assess progress toward weight loss, the nurse notes that the patient's diet is weighted heavily toward simple carbohydrates, the nurse should

a. advise the patient to eat more complex carbohydrates.
b. advise the patient to try to eliminate simple carbohydrates.
c. refer the patient to a nutritionist.
d. advise the patient to eat more protein and fats.

108. If a patient with chronic constipation finds that, when her constipation worsens, she has occasional urinary incontinence, the MOST appropriate referral is to

a. gastroenterologist.
b. urologist.
c. nutritionist.
d. internist.

109. If a patient usually has decaffeinated tea, orange juice, eggs, toast, and bacon for breakfast but finds that urinary incontinence increases after breakfast, the patient should be advised to skip the

a. tea.
b. eggs.
c. bacon.
d. orange juice.

110. If a patient has developed increasing urinary incontinence and the caregiver request that a Foley catheter be inserted to make care easier, the caregiver should be advised that the primary reason that Foley catheters are avoided in patients is because of

a. increased cost.
b. risk of infection.
c. risk of bladder perforation.
d. risk of urethral trauma/ulcerations.

111. If a patient has a temporary indwelling catheter following surgery to relieve incontinence, how frequently should the drainage bag be emptied?

a. every 2 to 3 hours
b. every 4 to 6 hours
c. every 8 to 9 hours
d. every 10 to 12 hours

112. Which of the following foods/beverages is indicated to help to keep the urine acidified?

a. orange juice
b. milk
c. grapefruit
d. cranberry juice

113. If a nurse is teaching a patient to do clean intermittent catheterization, after gathering supplies and washing hands, the next step should be to

a. locate the meatus by touch or with a mirror.
b. spread the labia and cleanse area with soap and water.
c. palpate the bladder.
d. lubricate the catheter with water soluble gel.

114. If a patient had a successful sling procedure to control urinary incontinence but is still so fearful of recurrence that she refuses to leave her home for any social activities and has become increasingly withdrawn and anxious, the nurse should recommend

a. referral to a psychologist.
b. meditation.
c. relaxation exercises.
d. discussion with urologist.

115. Which of following is appropriate when carrying out pelvic floor muscle assessment for a female patient?

a. position patient supine with feet in stirrups
b. position the patient in left Sims position
c. position the patient in semisupine position with hips and knees flexed
d. maintain separation of the patient's feet during the procedure

116. If a 15-year-old patient with a spinal cord injury has a nursing diagnosis of "impaired urinary elimination related to reflex incontinence" and interventions include teaching the patient to carry out intermittent self-catheterization, the expected outcome would be

a. positive self-image.
b. catheterization.
c. knowledge: treatment procedure.
d. self-care toileting.

117. What is a good strategy for helping an elderly female patient overcome feelings of low self-esteem related to chronic illness, overactive bladder, and loss of autonomy?

a. praise the patient constantly for any activities
b. tell the patient she has no reason to feel so depressed
c. provide opportunities for the patient to make decisions
d. encourage the patient to focus on positive factors

118. Docusate sodium (Colace®) relieves constipation by

a. increasing fecal bulk
b. increasing absorption of water and fat.
c. preventing reabsorption of water and adding lubrication.
d. stimulating muscle contractions/peristalsis.

119. If a caregiver complains about the odor of a home patient's bedside commode, the best suggestion is to

a. clean and leave a small amount of water and disinfectant in the bottom of the bucket.
b. use spray air fresheners each time the patient uses the commode.
c. place the commode outside periodically to air out.
d. replace the bucket periodically if it has an odor.

120. If a caregiver has used zinc oxide ointment to protect a patient's skin from urine and feces, the BEST way to remove the ointment is with

a. soap and water.
b. cleansing wipes.
c. mineral oil.
d. alcohol wipes.

Answers and Explanations

1. D: Bethanechol is sometimes prescribed to patients with detrusor underactivity, such as associated with diabetic neuropathy, because it stimulates muscarinic receptors in the detrusor muscle, causing it to contract and helping to facility bladder emptying. Bethanechol also increases peristalsis in the GI system, so it may cause diarrhea. Other adverse effects include excess salivation, dizziness, orthostatic hypotension, headache, nausea, and vomiting. The drug should not be given to those with asthma, hyperthyroidism, heart disease, bradycardia, and Parkinson's disease. Bethanechol is advised for short-term use only.

2. B: In order to prevent migration of bacteria and urethral trauma from the weight of a full urine bag, the drainage bag should be emptied every 4 to 6 hours; however, in many facilities, routine emptying occurs at the ends of shifts—every 8 to 12 hours—putting the patient at increased risk of infection. Drainage bags should not be emptied into measuring containers used by different patients because of the risk of cross contamination, and the drainage spout should be cleansed with an alcohol swab before opening and after draining.

3. D: The most common self-care method both males and females use to manage urinary incontinence is limiting fluid intake; unfortunately, this increases the risk of urinary infection and constipation, which may worsen urinary incontinence. Other commonly used self-care methods include defensive urination (urinating on a frequent schedule or before activities), toilet mapping (searching and finding the location of toilets), wearing absorptive pads (especially women), and limiting activities, sometimes to the point of remaining essentially homebound.

4. A: Once a fecal impaction has been identified (usually through symptoms and digital exam), the initial step is to administer a warm oil retention enema to soften the stool and provide lubrication. This is followed by manual removal in which the nurse uses a finger to break up the mass of stool. Stimulant suppositories may be used once the stool is broken up to help with expulsion, and a soapsuds enema may help to empty the rectum and stimulate contractions.

5. C: Atrophic vaginitis is common in older adults, occurring in up to 40%, because of decrease in estrogen following menopause. Atrophic vaginitis is characterized by vaginal itching, soreness, burning and dyspareunia. The vulva and vaginal mucosa are atrophic with the mucosa appearing dry and pale or red and ecchymotic. The tissue bleeds easily and may show slight ulcerated areas. Discharge varies but usually is scant and may be blood-tinged because of mucosal irritation. Atrophic vaginitis increases risk of urinary tract infections. Treatment includes transvaginal estrogen and lubricants.

6. B: Rectosigmoidal outlet delay constipation often responds well to biofeedback, which helps the patient learn to relax the muscles of defecation. Typically, the patient cannot adequately relax the puborectalis muscle and the external anal sphincter, resulting in inhibited defecation or defecation prolonged longer than 10 minutes with reduced frequency to sometimes less than 3 times weekly, so stool is often very hard. When the patient strains, the levator ani muscle does not relax, resulting in complete or partial blockage. Patients often assist defecation by splinting the anus.

7. A: Patients who have chronic constipation and must strain to defecate have increased risk of urinary tract infections and prolapse of pelvic organs. Chronic straining can impair neurological function, effecting both bladder and bowel function because of the close proximity of the organs. Chronic constipation also contributes to urinary retention and incontinence, primarily stress incontinence, possibly because of damage to pelvic floor muscles from straining. Studies have found that treating constipation can also reduce urinary frequency and urgency.

8. D: During the initial trial period of 3 days, the first intervention is to ask patients if they are wet or dry to help them focus attention on what it feels like, to check, and then provide feedback. Then, patients should be asked if they want to use the toilet and prompted 3 times if they refuse. Patients should be assisted to the toilet and encouraged to urinate. After the initial period, scheduled verbal reminders and positive feedback should be provided.

9. B: A few times a week (score 3) and small splashes (score 2) correspond with a moderate ranking. Frequency is multiplied by quantity of incontinence to arrive at the score. Frequency: (1) less than 1 time monthly, (2) a few times monthly, (3) a few times weekly, (4) every day/night. Quantity: (1) drops, (2) small splashes, (3) larger volume. Based on the scores, the severity is classified as:

- 1 to 2: Slight.
- 3 to 6: Moderate.
- 8 to 9: Severe.
- 12: Very severe.

10. B: While all of these are risk factors for fecal incontinence, the primary risk factor is institutionalization of the elderly, for a variety of reasons. Patients often receive medications that are constipating, their diets may be lacking in adequate fiber, their disease may impair bowel function, they may not drink adequate fluids, their activity may be limited, and they may need to delay toileting if no one is available to assist them or if their mobility is impaired.

11. D: Stroke is a risk factor for urge incontinence. About 40% of patients with strokes suffer from urinary incontinence. Other risk factors for urge incontinence include diabetes mellitus (especially if it is poorly controlled), neurological diseases (MS and Parkinson's disease), and advanced age. Vaginal delivery, chronic cough (such as associated with asthma or COPD), and obesity are all risk factors for stress incontinence. Debilities of age and dementia are most commonly associated with functional incontinence.

12. A: Problems with the bladder may be categorized as those related to storage, emptying, or mixed storage and emptying problems. Acute and chronic retention with or without overflow incontinence are problems with emptying of the bladder. Problems with storage include those related to bladder dysfunction (such as urge incontinence), those associated with impairment of sphincter function (such as stress incontinence), and other dysfunctions (such as extra-urethral urinary incontinence, and functional incontinence). Mixed problems include neurogenic dysfunction (reflex incontinence).

13. B: The bladder of an adult can usually hold 300 to 600 mL of urine. A distended bladder may hold more urine, but distention increases the risk of reflux, incontinence, and bladder rupture. If the bladder is distended and painful, then catheterization may be necessary if the patient is unable to urinate. The body of the bladder is comprised of the smooth detrusor muscle, which can distend to accommodate urine and then contract to expel the urine.

14. C: In older adult females, prevalence of stress urinary incontinence decreases and urge urinary incontinence increases with overall prevalence of incontinence doubling between ages 50 to 70 with up to a third of females experiencing some form of urinary incontinence between ages 80 to 90 although males have even higher rates of urinary incontinence, with prevalence tripling between ages 50 to 70. Additionally, functional incontinence is an increasing problem as people age and disease or mobility impairment interferes with toileting.

15. B: Rectocele: Prolapse of the posterior vaginal wall with the rectum can result in constipation and fecal incontinence. Rectal prolapse: Prolapse of the everted rectum through the anus results in difficulty with defecation. Enterocele: Prolapse of the proximal vagina and small intestine against the posterior vaginal wall results in pelvic pressure, backache (relieved by lying down), and difficulty defecating. Cystocele: Prolapse of the anterior vaginal wall with the bladder can result in urge incontinence and dysuria.

16. D: Some pessaries are intended for self-care, and can be removed daily, weekly, monthly, (depending upon the type) washed with soap and water, and reinserted. Others are removed, cleansed, and reinserted periodically by a health care provider. In general, pessaries should not be left in place for more than 4 months at a time to ensure that there are no complications. While the pessary does not cure pelvic organ prolapse, it may alleviate symptoms. Some women use a pessary for many years and require no other treatment. Others use it temporarily while awaiting surgical repair.

17. C: Because of age and frailty, this patient is a poor candidate for surgical repair, so a ring pessary, which is used for first- and second-degree uterovaginal prolapse is indicated. Hodge pessary is used for mild cystocele and cube pessaries for third-degree uterovaginal prolapse. Pessaries are plastic or silicone removable prosthetic devices that are placed in the vagina for management of pelvic muscle support defects, such as cystocele and rectocele. They are also frequently used for stress incontinence.

18. D: The best solution is probably to get the patient up for scheduled toileting at midnight since the patient urinates on a fairly regular schedule at night. Nocturia is common with older males, so restricting fluids alone may not alter the pattern. Alzheimer patients who are active often remove disposable undergarments or become even more confused when trying to urinate, and disposable undergarments should be reserved for incontinence. Patients with dementia will usually not remember to use a urinal.

19. A: The timed up and go (TUG) evaluates the time a patient requires to stand from a chair with armrests, walk 3 meters, turn, return, and sit back down. Those requiring more than 14 seconds are at risk for falls. The Katz ADL test evaluates normal activities, such as bathing, dressing, transferring, walking, using the toilet, grooming, and eating and includes timed tests for various activities. Instrumental Activities of Daily Living evaluates ADLs as well as ability to manage affairs (including finances), arrange transportation, use prosthetic devices, shop, and telephone. Functional Ability Rating Scale evaluates limitations in major life activities, such as self-care, communication, self-direction, ability to live independently, learning, and ability to handle economic affairs.

20. D: When fitting a penile sheath, the most important measurement is the penile circumference. If the circumference is too small, it can result in constriction and impaired circulation while if it is too big, folds may occur that result in leakage. The retracted penile length should be measured with the patient standing and sitting because a length of less than 5cm may require a shorter length device. If the penis retracts completely, then the penile sheath is contraindicated. The flaccid penile length is usually measured except for patients with spinal cord injuries who have spontaneous erections.

21. C: Vesicles are serous fluid-filled blisters between skin layers up to 0.5 cm in diameter, such as those associated with herpes simplex, and are superficially elevated. Bullae are similar in appearance to vesicles but larger than 0.5 cm in diameter, such as with second-degree burns. Papules are elevated lesions up to 0.5 cm in diameter, such as nevi. Macules are small, flat lesions that can be seen but not palpated, such as petechiae. Pustules are superficially elevated pus-filled lesions, such as impetigo.

22. A: Ureteral ectopia occurs when a ureter (usually a duplicate) implants at a site other than the bladder. In males, the most common implantation site is the urethra while in females it is the urethra or vagina. When a ureter is implanted in the vagina, then the patient experiences vaginal leakage of urine, which can be misdiagnosed as urinary incontinence. Treatment varies from none (if no symptoms are present) to surgical repair, with the type of surgery depending on whether the ureter is a duplicate or not.

23. D: Urination by classic reflex mechanism occurs in neonates and infants. Bladder distention sends messages via stretch receptors to the brain and spinal reflex mechanism, resulting in contraction of the bladder and urination. Bladder capacity remains very limited for the first half year of life, so the infant usually urinates about 20 times daily; however, then frequency usually begins to decrease. Infants are usually not consciously aware of bladder filling until between 12 and 24 months.

24. B: The most significant factor in changes in male urinary sphincter function is benign prostatic hypertrophy. Benign prostatic hypertrophy/hyperplasia usually does not develop until after age 40 but results from the second growth phase that begins at about age 25. The prostate may slowly enlarge, but the tissue encapsulating it restrains outward growth, so the gland compresses the urethra. The bladder wall also goes through changes, becoming thicker and irritated, so that it begins to spasm, causing frequent urinations. The bladder muscle eventually weakens and the bladder fails to empty completely.

25. C: Hydrocele is a collection of fluid that is circumscribed and usually found in the tunica vaginalis of the testis or along the spermatic cord. It feels soft on palpation and allows the examining finger above the mass and transilluminates. Varicocele, varicose veins of the spermatic cord, is most often felt on the left side and feels separate from the testis. Epidermoid cysts are small (less than 1cm), firm, yellow, and nontender and usually are multiple. Scrotal hernia, usually an indirect inguinal hernia, does not allow the examining finger above it.

26. B: The rounded posterior surface of the prostate gland is palpated rectally through the anterior rectal wall, so any lesions in the anterior area of the prostate are not palpable. The normal prostate gland is about 2.5 cm in length. A hard area on the prostate may indicate a cancerous lesion. A symmetrically enlarged prostate usually indicates benign prostatic hypertrophy. If the prostate is swollen and very tender to palpation, the patient may have acute prostatitis.

27. A: The best schedule for changing indwelling catheters is as needed by the individual patient based on problems associated with the catheter, such as encrustation and signs of urinary infection, rather than the routine change every 3 to 4 weeks that is common practice (usually because of insurance coverage rules). Some patients routinely develop encrustations or blockage and should have more frequent catheter changes to avoid trauma while others may safely go up to 6 weeks between catheter changes.

28. D: The best time to take a loop diuretic to prevent nocturia is about 6 hours before bedtime. Diuretics are a leading cause of urinary incontinence, especially in older adults. Most people take diuretics in the early morning, assuming the effects will lessen by bedtime, but diuretics increase thirst and fluid intake, and this combined with increased production of urine during the night often results in nocturia two or three times, so taking the diuretic much later in the day can often reduce nocturia.

29. C: Hesitancy is difficulty starting urine flow and delayed onset of urine flow after the person attempts to urinate. Intermittent stream is unintentional starting and stopping of urine flow while urinating. Poor stream is reduced force of urine flow and prolonged urine flow (occurs primarily in males). Straining is the need to utilize intra-abdominal pressure by bearing down with a Valsalva maneuver strongly to begin, maintain, or increase urine flow although this maneuver can increase the risk of prolapse if it occurs over an extended time period.

30. A: Although both urinary and fecal incontinence can have a profound effect on the quality of life, many patients are embarrassed to broach the subject with health care providers. Some patients actively try to conceal their problem because they fear others will view them negatively. Many patients try to deal with incontinence with self-care strategies, and it's not uncommon for patients to experience incontinence for a number of years before seeking professional help. Depression associated with incontinence may further prevent people from discussing the problem with healthcare providers.

31. D: The Bristol Stool Form has descriptions and pictures to help people identify the correct type of stool.

- *Type 1*: Separate small hard lumps of stool that are difficult to pass.
- *Type 2*: Sausage-shaped lumpy stool.
- *Type 3:* Sausage-shaped and lumpy but with cracks on the surface.
- *Type 4:* Long, smooth, soft, snake-like stool.
- *Type 5*: Soft blobs of stool that are easily passed and have clear-cut edges.
- *Type 6*: Mushy, fluffy pieces of stool with uneven ragged edges.
- *Type 7:* Watery stool that is entirely liquid.

Bowel diary should include time of each event (defecation, incontinence, and flatus), type of stool, amount, activity at the time of incontinence, intake of food and drinks, and all medications.

32. B: Contained incontinence means that the patient must use absorbent products or other materials to contain urinary leakage and is not able to remain continent with or without the help of caregivers. This is the most common type of incontinence, especially among older adults, who frequently depend on absorbent products. In some cases, patients may gain partial continence through scheduled toileting and the use of medications, but the patients must use absorbent products because some incontinence remains.

33. C: While in the early stages of MS frequency, urgency, and urge incontinence are common, over time almost all patients develop neurogenic bladder and long-term urinary retention. The most common treatment is clean intermittent catheterization although as the disease progresses some patients will require catheterization with continuous drainage, especially when they can no longer do catheterizations independently. Baclofen is sometimes useful with mild urinary retention but not with advanced disease. The nerves that control bowel movements can also be affected, causing constipation and fecal incontinence.

34. D: The "knack" is a preventive use of Kegel exercises. Women are taught to contract the pelvic floor muscles right before and during events that usually cause stress incontinence. For example, if a woman feels as though she is going to sneeze, she immediately contracts and holds the pelvic floor muscles and until the sneeze is over. This contraction provides additional support to the proximal urethra, helping to keep the sphincter closed. The "knack" is particularly useful if used before and during stress events, such as coughing, sneezing, lifting, standing, swinging a golf club, or laughing.

35. B: Because the urethral insert must be removed in order to urinate, it is not useful for extended time periods, so the best use is during specific activities that cause stress incontinence, such as playing tennis. Urethral stents are disposable tampon-like devices that are inserted into the urethra with an applicator. Once inserted with the tip in the bladder, the balloon tip expands to create a seal that prevents urinary leakage. Patients should cleanse the genital area before insertion and use clean technique to decrease risk of infection.

36. C: Vaginal weights/cones are most effective as part of the treatment regimen for stress incontinence because they help strengthen pelvic floor muscles. The weights are cone-shaped with a string attached to help with removal. The patient initially inserts the lightest weight and does exercises contracting and relaxing the pelvic floor muscles for at least 15 minutes twice daily. When the patient is able to hold a weight in place for a minute, she increases to the next size.

37. A: During digital evaluation of the pelvic floor muscles, one (for some nulliparous women) or two fingers (for multiparous women) are inserted into the vagina and the woman asked to tighten the muscles to squeeze the fingers. If no response is felt, then the nurse should press lightly against the posterior vaginal wall and have the patient try again. If the nurse feels contraction, the patient should be asked to repeat the contractions a number of times, with the nurse providing feedback.

38. A: Intrinsic urethral sphincter dysfunction (ISD) usually requires surgical intervention, such as periurethral injection or suburethral sling, to reduce urinary leakage. Patients with severe stress incontinence and a Q-tip test with a straining angle less than 30 degrees should be further evaluated for ISD. ISD occurs in both males and females and is characterized by increased incontinence when the patient is standing (gravitational incontinence). ISD is common after prostatectomy and TURP. The bladder neck and proximal urethra function poorly in ISD.

39. B: When setting the amplitude (intensity of electrical current) for pelvic floor electrical stimulation, the amplitude should be gradually increased until an anal wink is observed. If no anal wink is noted, then the amplitude is not adequate for therapy. Other parameters that must be adjusted include ramping (typically set at 0.5 ramps), frequency rate (50 pulses per second for stress incontinence and 13 pulses per second for urge incontinence), and duty cycle (1:1 or 1:2).

40. D: Acidic urine is more resistant to infection, so urinary pH should not drop below 5. The most effective treatment is ascorbic acid 1 g daily or methenamine hippurate with ascorbic acid 1-2 g daily. Cranberry juice or cranberry tablets (300 to 400 mg BID) are also recommended for patients with catheters but for a different reason: The tannin found in cranberries interferes with bacterial adherence of *E. coli*, the most common cause of urinary infections.

41. A: Isolating the right muscles to tighten is important for pelvic floor muscle exercises. Tightening the stomach, leg, or other muscles is ineffective. Patients should not hold their breath during the exercises because this may tighten other muscles. Three methods, from easiest to most complex, include:

1. Stop flow of urine in the midst of urination. This is the easiest because a patient gets immediate feedback.
2. Pull in the anus as though trying to stop from passing flatus.
3. In supine position, place finger inside the vagina and squeeze as though trying to stop urine. Tightness should be felt.

42. C: A normal volume of voided urine for an adult is greater than 250 mL (300 to 600 mL) and the volume of residual urine should be less than 100 mL or one-quarter of total bladder volume. Measurement is typically done as part of urodynamic studies, such as uroflowmetry, which may be used as a baseline study for further evaluation. Once the patient has urinated and attempted to empty the bladder, then the residual capacity is assessed either with straight catheterization or with ultrasound bladder scan.

43. A: Up to 5% of males undergoing radical prostatectomy develop severe post-prostatectomy incontinence, generally because the urinary sphincter is injured during surgery, and the most effective option is the artificial sphincter, which places an inflatable silicone cuff about the urethra. The patient presses a valve to deflate the cuff, allowing urination. Up to 80% of males achieve continence with the device. The valve is left open for 6 to 8 weeks after surgery to allow healing. Permanent restrictions include riding bicycles, motorcycles, or horses. Other treatment options include injection of a bulking agent about the urethra and the urethral sling procedure.

44. B: Patients with diabetic neuropathy are most at risk for overflow urinary incontinence because nerve supply to the bladder, urethra, and pelvic floor muscles is impaired, and this results in reduced sensation of bladder fullness as well as urinary retention causing the detrusor muscle to over-distend so that bladder does not empty adequately. Both of these effects lead to overflow incontinence. Some diabetic patients may have detrusor overactivity as well with urgency, frequency, and urge incontinence.

45. A: Urge incontinence is usually treated with anticholinergics/antispasmodics, such as oxybutynin or tolterodine. Some medications, such as fesoterodine fumarate, specifically target overactive bladder. SSRIs, such as sertraline, may cause urinary frequency and incontinence although SNRIs, such as duloxetine, may be used for stress incontinence. Desmopressin is specifically used for urinary frequency and excessive thirst associated with diabetes insipidus although it may also be used as a treatment for bed-wetting.

46. B: A female patient doing clean intermittent catheterization (CIC) should initially insert the catheter two to three inches, guiding it upward until urine begins to flow, and then gently insert the catheter about another inch. The patient may sit on the toilet for the procedure, being sure to clean the vulva and urethral opening with soap and water or individually packaged wipes containing benzalkonium chloride, wiping from top to bottom. The catheter may be lubricated with water-soluble lubricant or water.

47. C: Anal manometry. Procedure:

- The lower bowel is cleansed, usually with Fleet enemas about 2 hours before the assessment and food is restricted during this time.
- With patient lying on left side, a balloon catheter is inserted into the rectum. A machine connects to the catheter to measure pressure.
- The balloon is inflated in the rectum to simulate a feeling of fullness and the need to defecate to test neurological response of the reflex pathways.
- Pressure measurements are taken while the patient tightens, relaxes, and pushes with the anal sphincter muscles, simulating holding stool and expelling stool.

48. A: Because patients may be embarrassed and uncomfortable discussing sexual functioning (especially with someone of the opposite gender), the PLISSIT model begins with asking the patient's permission to discuss sexual function. If the patient agrees, then the nurse can go to the next steps:

- P: Ask permission.
- LI: Provide limited information about sexual function.
- SS: Provide specific suggestions for dealing with sexual dysfunction.
- IT: Refer to a specialist in sex therapy for intensive therapy.

If the patient declines, the nurse should tell the patient that they can discuss it later if the patient changes his or her mind and ask if there is someone else with whom the patient would feel more comfortable discussing the issue.

49. D: With uroflowmetry, the explosive flow pattern often indicates stress incontinence although it is a normal flow pattern for some individuals, so further testing is indicated. The normal flow pattern is a Bell curve with maximum/peak flow of greater than or equal to 12 mL per second and average of greater than 8 mL per second. But the maximum/peak flow with an explosive flow pattern is often much higher, such as up to 35 mL or 40 mL per second flow, but the duration of urination is shorter, so the flow pattern is high and narrow.

50. B: During cystometry, fluid (NS or contrast material) is instilled into the bladder through a catheter, and the patient is asked to report sensations as the bladder fills:

- First sensation: Patient first begins to feel bladder pressure.
- First wish to urinate: Patient feels the need to urinate but is able to delay urination without fear of leakage.
- Strong wish to urinate: The patient feels a persistent need to urinate but is not afraid of leakage.
- Maximum cystometric capacity: The patient has a strong urge to urinate and cannot delay because of fear of leakage.

51. C: The purpose of assessing abdominal leak point pressure is to determine urethral sphincter competence. For the test, the bladder is filled with a set volume of fluid and the patient asked to bear down as though trying to urinate but with mild effort at first and progressing in increments until urinary leakage occurs, with the lowest pressure at which urinary leakage occurs recorded. Patients may be asked to cough or carry out the Valsalva maneuver to determine if abdominal stress results in incontinence. Normal sphincter activity is greater than 90 cm H_2O while less than 60 represents intrinsic sphincteric deficiency.

52. A: Patients undergoing sigmoidoscopy (rigid or flexible) usually require no or minimal sedation although patients with low pain threshold or severe anxiety may need moderate/conscious sedation. Moderate sedation (narcotic, such as fentanyl, and benzodiazepine, such as midazolam) is usually indicated for endoscopic procedures, such as upper endoscopy and colonoscopy. Procedures that are complicated or prolonged may require deep sedation with the same drugs as well as droperidol or propofol. General anesthesia is generally indicated only for complex and surgical procedures because of increased risks associated with general anesthesia.

53. A: A daily stool softener, such as Colace, may decrease fluid reabsorption and move stool through the colon more quickly. A bulk former, such as Metamucil, may also be helpful, but fiber has already been added to the diet without relieving the constipation. The patient should not routinely take laxatives as this may, in time, worsen constipation. Routine enemas of any kind should be avoided unless absolutely necessary to relieve impaction as they may cause loss of muscle tone and irritation of tissues.

54. C: Endoanal ultrasonography is most indicated for suspected of tearing, scar tissue, or other damage of the anal sphincters and may help to rule out other causes of incontinence. The ultrasound may be done endoscopically with the ultrasound probe on the end of the endoscope. The probe is inserted into the anus and pictures are taken. Usually no special preparation or follow-up is necessary for endoanal ultrasonography, and the procedure usually takes less than half an hour.

55. C: An older adult patient with hypomotility and reduced bowel transit time may not be a good candidate for a high fiber diet because stool moves through the colon more slowly than normal, allowing more reabsorption of fluid from the stool. Increasing fiber may, in this case, increase constipation and the risk of fecal impaction, especially if the patient has inadequate fluid intake. Bulk formers such as Metamucil should be used with care in older patients as well.

56. D: The KUB x-ray is often done as a survey to determine if size, shape, and location of organs are normal. KUB can also be helpful in identifying constipation and kidney stones since both of these will show up on x-ray. Fluid and air in the intestines may also be seen, and obstructed areas may appear as dilated. Abnormal lesions, such as tumors, or thickening of intestinal walls may be evident. KUB may help to determine what further tests are needed.

57. B: Oxybutynin TDS, the transdermal patch, should be applied 2 times weekly on the same days each week (such as Sunday and Wednesday), rotating to different sites on the hip, abdomen, or buttocks. The patch should not be exposed to sunlight, so it should be placed on clean, dry skin where it will be covered by clothing but not about the waistband or in an area where it may become dislodged. Patients can swim and shower with the patch but should avoid soaking in a tub for long periods or rubbing the patch while bathing.

58. D: Usually a renal ultrasound requires no fasting, but when the bladder is to be scanned, then the patient must have a full bladder before the exam. A typical prep is to drink adequate clear liquids the day prior to the test and at least 24 ounces of fluid in the morning before the test, finishing with the last of the liquid about one-half hour before the ultrasound begins to ensure that the bladder is full.

59. B: Because waist circumference is based on averages, the measurements won't hold true for females who are too far outside of average size, but generally a waist measurement greater than 35 inches is a risk factor for obesity-related health problems for females and greater than 40 inches for males. Waist measurements are often considered in relation to the BMI, with 25 to 29.9 overweight, 30-34.9 obese, 35 to 39.9 severely obese, and greater than 40 morbidly obese.

60. B: When patients do a 24- to 48-hour pad test at home, they carry out normal activities and save incontinence pads of known weight in sealed plastic bags so they can be weighed in the office; however, with an abbreviated one-hour test, the patient with a full bladder wears an incontinent pad and is asked to carry out a number of provocative activities, such as coughing and jumping. After an hour, the incontinent pad is removed and weighed.

61. A: When assessing the urethral pressure profile (UPP) during urodynamic studies, the urethral closure pressure is calculated by subtracting the intravesical pressure (P-ves) from the intraurethral pressure (P-ura). The urethral closure pressure is the fluid pressure needed to open a closed urethra. The maximum difference between the two measurements comprises the maximum urethral closure pressure (MUCP). An MUCP less than 20 cm H_2O is considered indicative of intrinsic urethral sphincter deficiency.

62. C: Transient urinary incontinence may result from many different factors, such as delirium, infection, atrophic vaginitis, medications, infection, depression, disease processes, constipation and fecal impaction, and impaired mobility, so the first step to determine the cause and then take measures to eliminate or control it. Treatment measures may include adjusting dosage of medications or administration time, or changing medications. Other measures include controlling constipation and disorders (such as diabetes and congestive heart failure), and modifying fluid intake.

63. D: The total recommended fluid intake from foods and fluids for an adult male is 3.7 L and for a female 2.7 L per day although this may vary somewhat according to age, condition, and size; however, much of this fluid is derived from foods, especially fruits and vegetables. Most people can use thirst as a guide to ensure adequate fluid intake, which should usually average 20 to 50 ounces daily. Water should comprise the majority of the fluid intake because many other fluids contain sodium, which affects fluid balance.

64. C: When double voiding, the patient urinates the first time and then remains seated at the toilet for a resting period of 2 to 10 minutes before urinating a second time. A second method involves urinating and then standing up (females) or stepping away (males) and then urinating a second time. Double voiding may be combined with Credé massage of the bladder if there is decreased outlet resistance although it may result in urinary reflux in some cases.

65. A: Smoking is associated with all types of urinary incontinence to some degree but especially with stress incontinence. Smoking often results in chronic cough, and coughing increases pressure on the pelvic floor and can result in damage to the pudendal and pelvic nerves. Smoking is a significant risk factor for bladder cancer and may also cause other lower urinary tract symptoms, such as frequency, incomplete bladder emptying, nocturia, and urgency. All patients should be advised to stop smoking.

66. B: Morbid obesity is a risk factor for stress incontinence as well as fecal incontinence, especially for the morbidly obese with a BMI greater than 30. Obesity causes increased pelvic pressure and impairment of muscles, nerves, and pelvic structures. Studies indicate that a loss of 5 to 10% of body weight often reduces prevalence of stress incontinence by at least 50% and that patients undergoing gastric bypass surgery often decreases prevalence of incontinence as people lose weight.

67. D: Habit training matches a toileting schedule to a patient's normal pattern (ascertained from a bladder diary), usually every 3 to 4 hours during the daytime hours. Patients should be asked to try to maintain the pattern and to delay toileting until the scheduled time unless the urge is unbearable. This type of training may be helpful for those with neurogenic bladder and those who are cognitively impaired. Habit training often requires the assistance of a caregiver, especially for cognitively impaired patients.

68. C: CAM: Assesses development of delirium. Factors indicative of delirium include:

- Onset: Acute change in mental status.
- Attention: Inattentive, stable or fluctuating.
- Thinking: Disorganized, rambling conversation, switching topics, illogical,
- Level of consciousness: Altered, ranging from alert to coma.
- Orientation: Disoriented (person, place, time).
- Memory: Impaired.
- Perceptual disturbances: Hallucinations, illusions.
- Psychomotor abnormalities: Agitation (tapping, picking, moving) or retardation (staring, not moving).
- Sleep-wake cycle: Awake at night and sleepy in the daytime.

MMSE and Mini-Cog are used to assess evidence of dementia or short-term memory loss, often associated with dementia of the Alzheimer type. GDS is self-assessment tool to identify older adults with depression.

69. A: While all of these may have some role in slowing progress of stool through the colon, the smooth muscle being less responsive to neural stimulation results in decreased peristalsis. While peristalsis is more active in the small intestine, it normally occurs in waves 2 or 3 times daily in the colon, so a decrease in peristalsis means that more fluid is reabsorbed from the fecal material, causing constipation. This is exacerbated by loss of elasticity in rectal walls and decreased strength and response of internal and external anal sphincters.

70. C: Because urge incontinency involves loss of bladder inhibition and increased urgency, incontinence may be triggered by such things as drinking water, listening to running water, or having the hands in water (such as when washing dishes). Additionally, patients often find that they are incontinent on the way to the toilet because the thought of urinating increases the urge. Patients with urge incontinence must usually wear incontinent pads of some type and often modify fluid intake during activities.

71. B: The most likely cause of a urine culture report indicating multiple organisms is specimen contamination. This can occur at any point in the collection and processing, so patients should be carefully instructed about the correct method of cleansing the tissue and obtaining a midstream urine sample. If a patient is catheterized, the sample must be taken directly from the catheter and not the drainage bag, which may be contaminated. Usually cultures showing an organism with a colony count of greater than 100,000 for a single organism indicate infection although colony counts of *E. coli* may cause infection with counts about one-tenth that.

72. D: The perimenopause phase of the reproductive system can begin in the latter part of the 30s or early 40s. Initially, one of the changes is a shorter menstrual cycle. The character of the menstrual flow may change also and periods may become quite irregular. The average age of menopause is about 51, but some women experience menopause in the 40s. As menopause approaches, estrogen levels decrease, ovulation ceases, and vaginal tissues may begin to show signs of atrophy.

73. D: The most common side effect of antimuscarinic drugs is dry mouth with constipation the next most common. CNS effects, such as drowsiness, dizziness, and blurred vision, are much less common. Patients receiving antimuscarinic drugs should be advised to sip fluids frequently and suck on hard candy to alleviate dry mouth. They should be advised regarding dietary management of constipation (such as adding prune juice and yogurt) and some may need to take stool softeners.

74. D: Patients who are incontinent of large amounts of urine and feces, especially those who are bedridden, usually require superabsorbent disposable adult diaper-like briefs. Reusable protective underwear is not convenient because of the need for frequent washing and drying and handling of soiled garments. Disposable underpads won't keep the upper bedding from being saturated and usually only contain a thin layer of absorbent material although they are frequently used in addition to adult diaper-like briefs.

75. A: Zinc oxide generally provides better protection from irritants although it is difficult to remove. This type of barrier is frequently used with patients who are incontinent to prevent incontinence dermatitis, which can deteriorate into pressure injuries. Moisture barrier pastes, many containing zinc oxide, are ointments with powder added to improve absorption and make them more durable and solid, providing a thick skin barrier. Barrier ointments/pastes are usually reapplied with each diaper change.

76. C: Between 20 and 30 injections of botulinum toxin A (BTX-A) are usually made into the bladder wall to treat bladder overactivity. BTX-A is a neurotoxin that inhibits release of acetylcholine to reduce detrusor contractions. The procedure is usually done on an outpatient basis with a cystoscope and local anesthetic. Side effects are usually minimal although detrusor underactivity with resultant urinary retention can occur, so post-void residual urines should be assessed after injections. Systemic reactions, such as respiratory compromise, are rare but can occur.

77. D: The bran-containing constipation recipe is made with one cup each of oat or wheat bran (unprocessed) and applesauce mixed with three-quarters cup of prune juice. The mixture may be stored in the refrigerator or freezer. Patients usually take 1 to 2 tablespoons of the mixture every evening along with a full glass of liquid. Constipation usually begins to abate within about 2 weeks but if not, then the dosage should be doubled. This recipe is frequently used in convalescent care and long-term care facilities.

78. A: Catheter-associated urinary infection (CAUTI) is the most common nosocomial infection and can lead to sepsis. CAUTI occurs in most patients with long-term catheters once or twice yearly, sometimes requiring hospitalization. While most non-catheter-associated urinary infections involve primarily one organism (such as *E. coli*), CAUTI often involves multiple organisms, some antibiotic resistant. Common CAUTI organisms include *Klebsiella, Proteus,* and *Enterobacter.* Antibiotic resistant organisms include *Pseudomonas aeruginosa*, *Candida albicans,* vancomycin-resistant *Enterococcus* and methicillin-resistant *Staphylococcus aureus.*

79. B: With normal urination, the first sensation of the need to urinate should occur when the bladder is about half full. The normal urination cycle includes:

1. Bladder filling with relaxation of detrusor muscle and contraction of pelvic floor muscles and urethral sphincter.
2. First sensation of urge to urinate occurs.
3. Bladder is full and desire to urinate causes detrusor muscle to contract and pelvic floor muscles and sphincter to relax (voluntary control).
4. Urination.

80. D: Although in general women are twice as likely to develop urinary incontinence as males, there are ethnic differences in prevalence rates. Caucasian women have the highest rate of stress incontinence probably because Caucasians tend to have weaker pelvic floor muscles and their bladder neck is lower than other groups. African American women have the lowest rates of stress incontinence but higher rates of both urge urinary incontinence and mixed urinary incontinence than women of other ethnic groups.

81. D: If using vaginal weights as part of pelvic floor muscle training, the weights should be held in place for up to 15 minutes BID. Holding them in place for longer periods may result in irritation to the tissues and muscle fatigue. Vaginal weights are generally cone shaped with a string attached (like a tampon) to facilitate removal and should be washed and dried between uses to reduce risk of infection. The patient starts with the lightest weight and when she can hold that in place for at least 15 minutes, she can move to the next size.

82. C: When educating a patient about medications, the nurse should advise the patient that the most common adverse effect of anticholinergic/antimuscarinic drugs is dry mouth and constipation. Less common adverse effects vary depending on the specific drug and age and condition of the patient but may include dyspepsia, increased intraocular pressure, cardiac disturbance, delirium/confusion, somnolence, and headache.

83. A: If an older male patient has been using curved leaf incontinent pads for mild urinary incontinence but complains that they won't stay in place and sometimes fall out, the nurse should ask the patient, "What style of underwear do you wear?" Older males often prefer boxer shorts because they are more comfortable, but there is not enough support to hold the incontinent pads securely. Snug fitting briefs are necessary to hold the incontinent pads in place.

84. B: The type of support group that is likely to be the most acceptable to the majority of patients who are referred for fecal incontinence is a gender specific group. Patients often feel shame and embarrassment about fecal incontinence and the stigma attached and are reluctant to discuss the issue with others, especially those of the opposite gender. Additionally, females and males may have to deal with different issues that can be difficult for patients to discuss in a mixed group.

85. A: Antiglycemic drugs, such as metformin, gliclazide, and acarbose (which are used in the treatment of diabetes type 2) may cause the patient to have loose stools and diarrhea, and if the patient also has poor sphincter control, this can contribute to fecal incontinence. Patients may need to change to other medications or reduce the dosage of existing medications. About 1 in 10 patients taking metformin develop GI problems, including diarrhea.

86. C: A contraindication to the use of a fecal pouch is ambulatory status. The pouch is used for patients who are non-ambulatory and need assistance to move up and down in the bed because doing so independently could dislodge the appliance. The skin to which the pouch is attached must be intact and clear of irritation. A skin barrier is usually applied to the skin and then the pouch applied by a bendable wafer that allows it to fit about the anus. Many pouches have a sealable port at the bottom so that the pouch can be emptied without removing the appliance.

87. A: An emollient (lanolin, petrolatum, liquid paraffin) forms a lipid barrier to protect skin against loss of water while a humectant (urea, clycerole, lactic acid) attracts moisture to the skin. Hydrating agents serves as oil repellents while anti-inflammatory agents reduce response to irritants. Skin products often contain a mixture of emollients, humectants, hydrating agents and anti-inflammatory agents, and the balance depends on the overall effectiveness of the product.

88. D: If a patient has involuntary loss of flatus, mucus, and feces without sensation or urge, this type of incontinence is classified as passive anal incontinence. Classifications:

- Fecal incontinence: Loss of feces.
- Mucus incontinence: Loss of mucus.

- Flatus incontinence: Loss of flatus.
- Anal incontinence: Loss of feces, mucus, and flatus.

Subtypes of each of the above include:

- Urge: Feels sensation of urgency.
- Passive: Feels no sensations.
- Functional: Unable to get to toilet because of barriers.

89. B: When beginning percutaneous tibial nerve stimulation and adjusting the setting, if the great toe dorsiflexes at a setting of 12, the setting of 11 (one below) should be used for the treatments, which usually take place for 30 minutes one time weekly for about 12 weeks. The setting is adjusted after the needle electrode and the surface electrode are in place. The needle electrode must be placed at a 60-degree angle to the skin. If there is no response to increased settings, the needle electrode must be removed and placed in a different spot.

90. C: If a patient has an artificial anal sphincter and deflates the balloon to have a bowel movement, the sphincter will automatically refill after 10 minutes. For the artificial sphincter, an inflatable sphincter is inserted about the anus with a pump implanted in the labia or scrotum. The pump can inflate and deflate the sphincter. When the patient has the urge to defecate, the sphincter is deflated and can be manually reinflated or automatically reinflated. This surgical procedure does not have a high success rate because of the potential for complications.

91. A: If, following a stroke, a patient has some residual paralysis and has difficulty cooking foods, engaging in recreational activities, dressing, and toileting independently, the referral that is most indicated is occupational therapy. The occupational therapist can evaluate the patient's needs and help the patient to develop compensatory strategies and can recommend appropriate assistive devices, such as the self-wipe bathroom toilet aid, elevated toilet seat, and grab bars for the bathroom.

92. B: If a patient is incontinent of stool only when the stool is loose, the primary intervention is a bulking agent, such as Metamucil®. If the loose stools are associated with diarrhea, then the patient may also need to take loperamide to reduce frequency and liquidity of stools. Bulking agents are high in fiber and absorb fluid, which results in thickening of the fecal material and stools that are firmer.

93. D: Following injections of a tissue bulking agent (Solesta®) to control fecal incontinence, the patient should be advised to avoid hot baths and physical exercise for 24 hours and then avoid strenuous exercise for an additional week and manipulation of the anus for 4 weeks. Solesta in the form of gel with tiny microspheres (beads) is injected (4 injections at each treatment) into the proximal section of the anal canal in order to narrow the anus. Contraindications include active IBD, previous radiotherapy to the pelvic area, anorectal disorders, rectocele or rectal prolapse, and immunodeficiency.

94. C: Following prostatectomy, especially radical prostatectomy, male patients (6 to 8%) may experience urinary incontinence because the internal bladder neck sphincter is damaged or removed. Most patients regain continence within 6 to 12 months and may benefit from pelvic floor muscle exercises (Kegel) and biofeedback. If the problem does not resolve, surgical repair may be indicated, but it is delayed until at least 6 months after the prostatectomy.

95. A: Over two-thirds of patients with multiple sclerosis report bowel dysfunction, most often constipation, but about half of patients experience some degree of fecal incontinence. Interventions for incontinence include reducing intake of fiber and avoiding artificial sweeteners, dairy products, alcohol, and caffeine. Patients should also practice scheduled toileting after meals and may benefit from pelvic floor muscle exercises (Kegel).

96. B: If during the physical examination, the patient does not exhibit the anal wink, this indicates the need for a neurological exam. If this reflex is absent, it may be an indication that the reflex arc has been impaired by damage to the spinal cord or the nerve roots (S2-S4). The anal wink reflex is elicited by stroking the skin about the anus. Normally, this will cause the external anal sphincter to contract.

97. A: Anatomic capacity is the volume of urine that the bladder is physically able to contain. Functional capacity is the volume of urine that the bladder can contain before the person feels sensations of urgency. Residual capacity is the volume of urine that remains in the bladder after urination. Cystometric capacity is the volume of urine the bladder holds during urodynamic testing.

98. D: The primary treatment for sensory urinary urgency is behavior modification. Sensory urgency occurs when the patient feels a strong urge to urinate or intense pain with small volumes of urine in the bladder but does not have an overactive detrusor muscle although sensory urgency may be part of the continuum of overactive bladder. Because the detrusor muscle is not hyperactive with sensory urgency, incontinence is rare although it can occur.

99. C: When assessing the patient's bladder diary, the first thing that the nurse should verify is the patient's pattern of waking and sleeping because this is important when assessing nocturia as opposed to daytime urination. The patient may, for example, stay up at night and sleep during the daytime. The number of voidings in 24 hours and the voiding intervals as well as the frequency and pattern of urinary incontinence should be assessed.

100. B: An absent bulbocavernosus response in a male patient is generally indicative of denervation of the spinal cord roots (S2-S4). The response is elicited during the digital rectal exam. The examiner gently squeezes the glans penis while a finger remains in the rectum. If the response is positive, the anal sphincter contracts about the finger. For females, the procedure is similar but the clitoris is gently tapped. If a catheter is in place, the catheter should be gently pulled to apply pressure to the bladder neck.

101. B: Voiding intervals during waking hours should be at least 2 hours although many patients will have longer intervals. Voiding intervals should be calculated for both daytime hours and sleeping hours. Except during sleeping hours, the intervals should not exceed 4 to 6 hours. If the interval is short, treatment will focus on increasing the interval. If the interval is long, this suggests that the patient may have sensory impairment or obstruction.

102. D: The initial treatment of choice for children with nocturnal enuresis is an enuresis alarm. One type of alarm that is in common use has a fluid-sensitive pad that causes an alarm to ring with even a few drops of urine so that the child awakens and can go to the toilet to urinate. This may be combined with desmopressin to decrease urinary output if the alarm is not sufficient. A tricyclic antidepressant, usually imipramine, may be administered if other treatments are unsuccessful.

103. A: The most common reason for failure and ultimate removal of an artificial urinary sphincter is infection, erosion, or both. An artificial urinary sphincter is often implanted to control post-prostatectomy incontinence. If the implant becomes infected (most often from Gram-positive bacteria that are part of skin flora), it often needs to be removed. Additionally, the implant typically needs to be replaced after about 8 to 10 years because it may begin to malfunction.

104. D: Hirschsprung disease should be suspected if a neonate fails to pass meconium within 48 hours, by which 99% of neonates have done so (90% do so within 24 hours). Hirschsprung disease (congenital aganglionic megacolon) is failure of ganglion nerve cells to migrate to part of the bowel (usually the distal colon), so that part of the bowel lacks enervation and peristalsis, causing stool to accumulate and leading to distention and megacolon.

105. B: The nurse must respect the right of the patient, but when patient's choices are risky or self-destructive and may interfere with adequate treatment, the nurse's best approach is to address the behavior in a nonjudgmental but factual manner and offer resources, such as information about 12-step groups or smoking cessation. The patient has the right to self-determination, but the nurse has a responsibility to the patient's welfare.

106. C: If a male newborn has hypospadias (a congenital defect where the urethra opens onto the underside of the penis and not in its usual place at the tip), the neonate should be carefully examined for undescended testicles and inguinal hernia as these are the most common anomalies found in association with hypospadias. The neonate may also have chordee (curvature) of the penis. Surgical repair is usually indicated but is not emergent if the neonate is urinating without difficulty. Circumcision should be delayed as some tissue from the prepuce may be utilized during repair.

107. C: If, when reviewing a patient's food diary to assess progress toward weight loss, the nurse notes that the patient's diet is weighted heavily toward simple carbohydrates, the nurse should refer to the patient to a nutritionist. The patient needs a clear understanding of the role of simple carbohydrates in weight gain and the importance of a balanced nutritious diet. The food diary is a valuable tool for reviewing the patient's intake of food.

108. A: If a patient with chronic constipation finds that when her constipation worsens, she also has occasional urinary incontinence the most appropriate referral is to a gastroenterologist. This physician can help to find the cause of the chronic constipation and provide treatment. Constipation can increase pressure on the bladder, and this may result in urinary incontinence in some patients, so relieving the constipation may resolve or minimize the problem. The patient should also be instructed in pelvic floor muscle exercises.

109. D: If a patient usually has decaffeinated tea, orange juice, eggs, toast, and bacon for breakfast but finds that urinary incontinence increases after breakfast, the patient should be advised to skip the orange juice. The patient should avoid drinking large amounts at one time and substitute water for most other fluids. Citrus fruits are bladder irritants and may increase stimulation of the detrusor muscle. It is better for the patient to eat a piece of fruit than to drink the juice so that the acidic intake is less concentrated.

110. B: If a patient has developed increasing urinary incontinence and the caregiver requests insertion of a Foley catheter to make care easier, the primary reason to avoid a Foley catheter is because a catheter increases the risk of infection. Catheters pose a daily risk of infection of up to 7%. Foley catheter use should be limited to less than a week if at all possible and should not be used solely for incontinence unless the urine has caused severe skin breakdown.

111. B: If a patient has an indwelling catheter following surgery to relieve incontinence, the drainage bag should be emptied every 4 to 6 hours to avoid overfilling the bag because bacteria can migrate up the internal and external lumen on the catheter and cause a urinary tract infection. Additionally, if the tubing is not properly secured and looped, a very full drainage bag may apply excess traction to the catheter. The indwelling catheter should be removed as soon as possible.

112. D: Cranberry juice is a beverage that is indicated to help to keep the urine acidified. Other foods that acidify the urine include prunes, plums, and high protein foods. Acidic urine is more resistant to infection, so foods that keep the urine alkaline increase the risk of infection. Acidic foods, such as citrus and other fruits, do not make the urine more acid but, in fact, increase its alkalinity. Other foods that should be limited include dairy products.

113. B: If a nurse is teaching a patient to do clean intermittent catheterization, after gathering supplies and washing hands, the next step should be to spread the labia and cleanse the area with soap and water. Then, the patient locates the meatus either by touch or with the use of a mirror, lubricates the catheter with water soluble gel, and inserts the catheter into the meatus until urine flows freely. After the urine stops draining, the patient removes the catheter and discards (if disposable) or washes if reusable.

114. A: If a patient had a successful sling procedure to control urinary incontinence but is still so fearful of recurrence that she refuses to leave her home for any social activities and has become increasingly withdrawn and anxious, the nurse should recommend referral to a psychologist because the patient may need professional help to overcome the fear and anxiety about recurrence of incontinence. The experience of incontinence is very traumatizing for some patients.

115. C: When carrying out pelvic floor muscle assessment for a female patient, the patient is positioned in semisupine position with the hips (45 degrees) and knees (120 degrees) flexed, and (if possible) with the soles of the feet touching and the knees relaxed to the side (abducted). The index and middle finger of one hand are inserted into the vagina while the other hand rests on the abdomen to feel the abdominal muscles. The patient is asked to tighten the muscles around the fingers and to try to life up and inward while the nurse assesses the patient's ability to contract the pelvic floor muscles.

116. D: If a 15-year-old patient with a spinal cord injury has a nursing diagnosis of "impaired urinary elimination" related to reflex incontinence and interventions include teaching the patient to carry out intermittent self-catheterization, the expected outcome would be self-care toileting. The outcome is the result of the intervention (catheterization) and should relate directly to the nursing diagnosis. Positive self-image may relate to a different nursing diagnosis. Treatment procedures relate to medical treatments rather than ongoing management.

117. C: A good strategy for helping an elderly female patient overcome feelings of low self-esteem includes providing opportunities for the patient to make decisions. Other strategies include providing companionship and listening and encouraging the patient to express her feelings and concerns. Positive feedback and praise should be given when earned rather than praising everything. Telling the patient that she has no reason to be depressed will invalidate her feelings and further lower her self-esteem. Low self-esteem is common among older adults because they have to deal with so many losses. They may become depressed, passive, and dependent.

118. B: Docusate sodium (Colace®) relieves constipation by increasing absorption of water and fat so that the stool is softer. Stool softeners are well tolerated by most patients and are used primarily to prevent constipation and to prevent straining although they may be less effective than bulking agents. They may also reduce discomfort for those with anal fissures or hemorrhoids. If patients have impaired intestinal mobility, the stool softener may cause soft stool to accumulate.

119. A: If a caregiver complains about the odor of a home patient's bedside commode, the best suggestion is to clean the bucket promptly after use and to leave a small amount of water and disinfectant in the bottom of the bucket to prevent odor and make the bucket easier to empty and clean. Males may be encouraged to use a urinal to void. Urinals are also available for females, but they are difficult to use for patients with limited mobility.

120. C: If a caregiver has used zinc oxide paste to protect a patient's skin from urine and feces, the best way to remove the paste is with mineral oil. Zinc oxide paste is thick and adherent and difficult to remove with soap and water. The nurse should apply mineral oil and gently wipe the zinc oxide paste away, avoiding excess rubbing that may irritate the skin. Because the skin must be cleaned after each episode of incontinence, zinc oxide may not always be the best choice.

Share Your Story!

It's Your Moment, Let's Celebrate It!

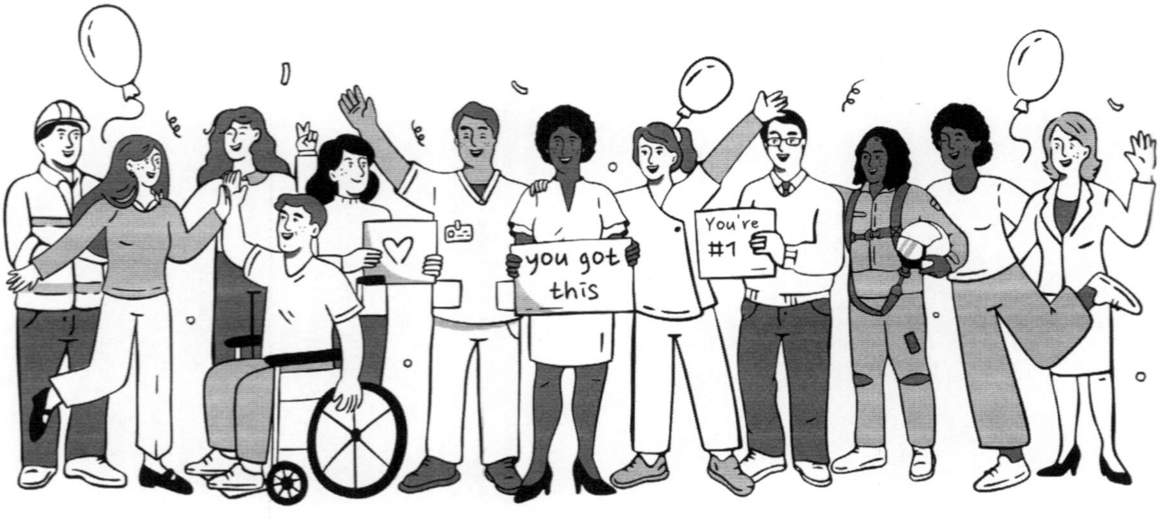

Share your story @mometrixtestpreparation